ENCYCLOPEDIA OF
FAMILY HEALTH

—— THIRD EDITION ——

ENCYCLOPEDIA OF
FAMILY HEALTH

—— THIRD EDITION ——

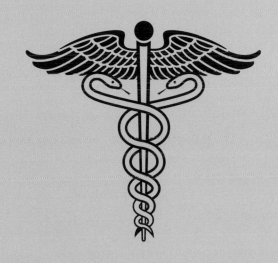

CONSULTANTS

David B. Jacoby, M.D.
Johns Hopkins School of Medicine

Robert M. Youngson, M.D.
Royal Society of Medicine

VOLUME 3

BRONCHITIS — COUNSELING

MARSHALL CAVENDISH
New York · London · Singapore

MEDICAL CONSULTANTS

Second Edition
David B. Jacoby, M.D.
Johns Hopkins School of Medicine
Associate Professor of Pulmonary and Critical
  Care Medicine

Third Edition
Robert M. Youngson, M.D.
Fellow of the Royal Society of Medicine
Officer of the Order of St John of Jerusalem
Diploma in Tropical Medicine and Hygiene
Fellow of the Royal College of Ophthalmologists

CONTRIBUTORS TO THIRD EDITION

David Arnot   Tom Jackson
Deborah Evans   Nathan Lepora
Leon Gray   Fiona Plowman
Joanna Griffin   Alison Tarrant
Tim Harris   Aruna Vasudevan
John Jackson

Picture Credits
(b – bottom; t – top; r – right; l – left; c – center)

Cover: Digital Vision: c; Dynamic Graphics: John Foxx & Images 4
Communication b/l, b/r; PhotoDisc: Don Farrall b/c, Keith Brofsky t/r.

American Cancer Society: 314, 316; Biophoto Associates: 332t, 400t; Brian
Nash: 321, 404, 405, 407, 408, 409, 410; C James Webb: 350, 338; Clarkes:
299; Corbis: Annie Griffiths Belt 301, Ariel Skelley 398, Bettmann 345, Brownie
Harris 313, Charles O'Rear 421, Jose Luis Pelaez 325, Laura Dwight 355t, 354,
LWA-Dann Tardif 393b, Norbert Schaefer 400b, Roy Morsch 419; Corbis Royalty
Free: 297, 381r; Corbis Saba: Najlah Feanny 377; Corbis Sygma: Dung Vo
Trung 302; Digital Vision: 402; Di Lewis: 310; Dudley Road Hospital:
Department of Medical Photographs 311; Frederick Mancini: 417, 422, 423b;
Getty Images: 323, 336, 355b, 357, 369, 397, 423t, Barros & Barros 429,
David Cornelius 334, David Harry Stewart 430, David Leahy 305, Steve Dunwell
333; Images: 390, 391; Imagingbody.com: 370, 403; Institute of Dermatology:
382; Institute of Ophthalmology: 327m, 416; Ken Moreman: 352; Kim Sayer:
306; M C Library: Alan Duns 366; Paul Brierley 389t; PhotoDisc: Doug Menuez
343, Jules Frazier 414, Keith Brofsky 312, 351, 361, 364, 412; Queen Mary's
Hospital, Roehampton: 401; Rex Features: A&M University 378, IPC
Magazines/Chat 413, Jeroen Oerlemans 380, Phanie Agency 427; Rousse
Laboratories Ltd: 393t; Sally & Richard Greenhill: 356; Science & Society Picture
Library: Health Education Authority 315; Science Photo Library: 327 m/l, Bsip
Bajande 340, CNRI 368, Custom Medical Stock Photo 322, Dr H C Robinson
361, Dr P Marazzi 319, Dr R Dourmashkin 396t & 396m, G-I Associates/Custom
Medical Stock Photos 387, H A Davies 349, Hank Morgan 425, John Greim 394,
428, Mark de Fraeye 358, 359, Peter Arnold/Szuson J Wong 360, Publiphoto
Diffusion/Ouellette & Theroux 363, Richard T Nowitz 395, Ron Sutherland
342m, Saturn Stills 367, 411, Sue Ford 328, University 'La Sapienza'
Rome/Professors P Motta & F Carpino 385, Wesley Bocxe 381l, Will & Deni
McIntyre 296, 335, 424; The Garden Picture Library: 309; Transworld Features:
342t; Vision International: CNRI 295, 339, 348, 389m, 375m 375b;
Westminster Children's Hospital: Dr H J Brueton 329; ZEFA: 353.

Marshall Cavendish
99 White Plains Road
Tarrytown, NY 10591-9001

www.marshallcavendish.com

© 2005, 1998, 1991 Marshall Cavendish Corporation

Library of Congress Cataloging-in-Publication Data

Encyclopedia of family health / David B. Jacoby, Robert M. Youngson.--
3rd ed.
              p. cm.
Includes bibliographical references and index.
      ISBN 0-7614-7486-2 (set)
      ISBN 0-7614-7489-7 (vol 3)
1. Medicine, Popular--Encyclopedias. 2. Health--Encyclopedias. 1. Jacoby,
David B. II. Youngson, R. M. III. Marshall Cavendish Corporation. IV. Title
RC81.A2E5 2004
610'.3--dc22   2003065554

Printed in China
08 07 06 05 04 5 4 3 2 1

Marshall Cavendish

Editor: Joyce Tavolacci
Editorial Director: Paul Bernabeo
Production Manager: Alan Tsai

The Brown Reference Group

Project Editor: Anne Hildyard
Editors: Jane Lanigan, Sally McFall
Designers: Jeni Child, Reg Cox, Karen Frazer
Picture Researcher: Clare Newman
Indexer: Kay Ollerenshaw
Illustrations: Samantha J. Elmhurst
Managing Editor: Tim Cooke
Art Director: Dave Goodman

CONTENTS

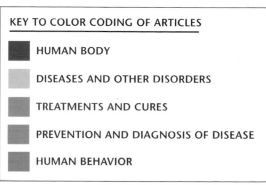

KEY TO COLOR CODING OF ARTICLES

■ HUMAN BODY

■ DISEASES AND OTHER DISORDERS

■ TREATMENTS AND CURES

■ PREVENTION AND DIAGNOSIS OF DISEASE

■ HUMAN BEHAVIOR

Bronchitis

Questions and Answers

I sometimes feel a little better after coughing in the morning. Since I am a heavy smoker, does that mean that I am in the early stages of bronchitis?

What you describe does not necessarily mean you have bronchitis, although smoking does contribute enormously to the disease. Some smokers believe that a morning cigarette will "cut the phlegm," but this is nonsense.

My uncle has difficulty in walking very far—even to the other end of the backyard. He blames this on his bronchitis. Is he right?

Yes. Generally, the worse the bronchitis, the less exercise the person can tolerate. Doctors divide bronchitis into four stages: one, a slight cough; two, breathlessness on exertion; three, breathlessness so severe that the patient is unable to leave the house; and four, breathlessness so severe that the patient is unable to converse normally.

Does bronchitis cause cancer?

No. But the smoking that often causes chronic bronchitis is a frequent cause of cancer. If you smoke more than 20 cigarettes a day, you increase your chance of developing lung cancer 20 times and your chance of getting chronic bronchitis 50 times.

If I give up smoking, will my chronic bronchitis get better?

It is possible that the course of the disease may be slowed and in some cases actually arrested by giving up smoking. However, chronic bronchitis is never reversed. Of course, your overall health will be improved by kicking the habit. Ask your family doctor for help. Nicotine gum and patches help some people to quit.

Bronchitis is a serious infection of the lungs and bronchial tubes, which can become chronic. Smoking cigarettes is mainly responsible, although other factors, such as breathing pollutants, can cause the condition.

Bronchitis is an inflammation of the main bronchial tubes—the bronchi—caused by a bacterial or viral infection (see Lung and Lung Diseases). It may develop suddenly, following a head cold (acute bronchitis), or it may persist or return regularly over many years, causing progressive degeneration of the bronchi and lungs (chronic bronchitis).

Certain people are more susceptible than others. Men are more likely to develop the condition than women, for example, outnumbering them 10 to one. The reasons for this are unclear. Smokers are 50 times more likely to get chronic bronchitis than nonsmokers.

Connection with smoking

Recent estimates suggest that 14.6 million Americans suffer from bronchitis and its common sequel, emphysema. These diseases together cause 70,000 deaths every year, making them the fifth most common cause of death in the United States. Eighty to 90 percent of cases are caused by cigarette smoking. The risk of death from bronchitis and emphysema is 30 times greater for people who smoke more than 25 cigarettes per day than for nonsmokers (see Emphysema).

In people who smoke, the probability of developing chronic bronchitis increases with age, and also with the number of cigarettes smoked. People who quit continue to have a greater liability to chronic bronchitis than nonsmokers, but this is less than if they were still smokers. This liability declines gradually with time. Cigar and pipe smokers also are liable to develop chronic bronchitis, but their risk is significantly lower than that of cigarette smokers.

A person with severe obstructive lung disease suffers from constant breathlessness, even at rest, is unable to undertake any exertion, and often has to use the neck and shoulder muscles in an exhausting attempt to get enough breath. Despite this, and although it may deprive them of up to 8 percent of the oxygen-carrying capacity of the blood, a sizable proportion of sufferers continue to smoke cigarettes. Generally bronchitis occurs with greater frequency in winter; in damp, cold climates; and in heavily polluted environments. Chilling, overcrowding, and fatigue are contributory factors.

Acute bronchitis is usually the result of a viral infection that spreads to the chest. Chronic bronchitis causes irritation and coughing. In this more serious form of bronchitis, the lungs lose their elasticity, and the exchange of vital oxygen, which is breathed in, and carbon dioxide waste, which is breathed out, is impaired. The bronchial tubes become permanently inflamed, and this inflammation results in an increased production of mucus from specialized cells in the walls of the bronchi, called goblet cells. The mucus coughed up is called sputum or phlegm.

Because it is difficult to look at the bronchi directly, doctors rely on the main symptom of the condition, phlegm production, to make a diagnosis. The color of the phlegm shows how serious the chronic bronchitis is.

HOW BRONCHITIC MUCUS AFFECTS THE RESPIRATORY SYSTEM

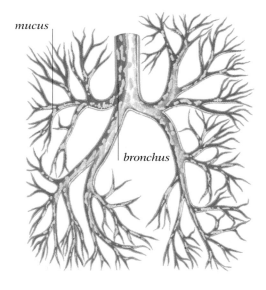

mucus

bronchus

▲ *Bronchitis causes increased production of mucus within the lungs.*

Symptoms

In acute bronchitis, the initial symptoms are a head cold, runny nose, fever and chills, aching muscles, and possibly back pain. This is followed by the most obvious symptom—a persistent cough. At first this is dry and racking, but later it becomes phlegmy. The cough is worse at night and if the person breathes smoke or fumes.

The main characteristic of chronic bronchitis is, again, a cough with phlegm, often occurring in paroxysms. Other symptoms depend on how much, or how little, emphysema is present. Emphysema causes the lungs to become overstretched, making breathing out difficult. A person with chronic bronchitis and no emphysema tends to be overweight and to have a bluish tinge to his or her lips. This is due to cyanosis, a bluish color in the blood caused by lack of oxygen (see Blood). In this case, shortness of breath occurs only during exercise. A person with bronchitis and a great deal of emphysema, on the other hand, has lost a lot of his or her oxygen-exchanging capacity. He or she will be short of breath at all times. People with both conditions tend to be underweight and, as the disease worsens, develop a barrel chest. The person with chronic bronchitis also wheezes.

Studies of autopsy findings from large numbers of people have shown that some discernible degree of emphysematous change is present in the lungs of 65 percent of men and 15 percent of women. However, only 1 percent of the population will develop sufficient emphysema to lead to symptoms and a clinical diagnosis. Clinical emphysema does not occur in nonsmokers, is present in 12 percent of people who have smoked less than one pack of cigarettes a day over a long period of time, and is present in nearly 20 percent of those who smoke one or more packs a day.

Treatment

The best treatment for acute bronchitis is bed rest in a warm room. Aspirin will reduce the fever, and cough medicines will relieve the cough. The sufferer may need antibiotics if the cause is bacterial.

Treatment of chronic bronchitis is more difficult because the patient's lungs are already damaged, and the obstruction of the airways is not easily reversible. The doctor may prescribe bronchial dilator drugs to relieve any such obstruction, while physical therapy will help the patient get rid of any phlegm.

Postural drainage can also be tried. This involves having the patient lie or sit in certain positions while the chest is tapped, causing the patient to cough up phlegm. Sitting at a 45-degree angle drains the upper chest; lying face up or face down with the chest above the head drains the middle and lower chest. In general, yoga and breathing exercises may ease shortness of breath. In severe cases, chronic bronchitis may require urgent hospital treatment. Oxygen might have to be given through the course of the illness.

The best form of relief for the condition is to remove bronchial irritants if possible. If the patient is a smoker, he or she should stop smoking immediately. Although chronic bronchitis cannot be reversed, it can be arrested. Sufferers should try to avoid environments where there are irritants, as these can bring on attacks.

Outlook

With acute bronchitis, the fever may last as long as five days and the coughing for weeks after that. However, provided that the patient receives treatment and takes sensible precautions, the illness will simply run its course, and the outlook is good.

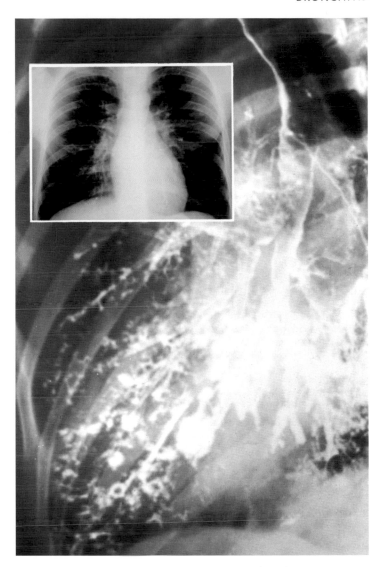

▲ *The alveoli in this lung of a person with chronic bronchitis are grossly swollen. A normal, clear lung is inset (left).*

Chronic bronchitis is more serious. It is a degenerative disease, particularly when combined with emphysema, and can result in death due to respiratory failure when there is insufficient oxygen in the blood. One of the most serious complications is carbon dioxide narcosis (stupor), together with increasing breathlessness, swollen ankles, and even heart failure.

The vital factor in the outcome of all cases of bronchitis is whether or not the passage of oxygen from the atmosphere to the blood becomes progressively obstructed. Such airflow obstruction, as it is called, occurs for two main reasons. First, persistent swelling of the linings of the air tubes in the lungs (because of inflammation) narrows them. Since many of the important smaller air tubes are no more than 0.039 inch (1 mm) in internal caliber, obstruction by edema (accumulation of fluid) can easily occur. Second, the total surface area available for the inward passage of oxygen and the outward passage of carbon dioxide becomes markedly reduced. Gas interchange in the lungs requires a very large surface area in the interface between the air and the blood. When large numbers of the tiny air sacs (alveoli) in the lungs break down to form larger spaces, a proportion of this surface is lost. This is what is called emphysema.

Questions and Answers

I have never smoked but have recently been diagnosed as having chronic bronchitis. Will this lead to emphysema?

No, that is not likely. Although chronic bronchitis is often caused and also made worse by smoking, it can be due to factors such as air pollution and industrial irritants. Clinical emphysema, by contrast, does not develop in nonsmokers. It occurs only in smokers, and the likelihood increases with the number of cigarettes smoked. The long-term effects of emphysema are present in 12 percent of those who smoke up to one pack a day, and in around 20 percent of those who smoke between one and two packs a day.

My uncle is constantly puffing on a pipe. Is it usual for pipe smokers to develop bronchitis?

People who smoke cigars and pipes are much less likely to develop chronic bronchitis than those who smoke cigarettes. However, if your uncle is worried, he should try and cut down on his pipe smoking. There is still some chance that he may develop bronchitis, or possibly mouth and lung cancers.

Is bronchitis a disease that can result in death?

Most definitely. In the United States, bronchitis ranks as the fifth most common cause of death, resulting in around 70,000 fatalities per year. Between 80 and 90 percent of all cases of the disease are caused by smoking. If you do not smoke, do not start; if you do smoke, quit.

My sister has bronchitis. Would she be able to borrow my asthma inhaler in an emergency?

Many people with bronchitis are prescribed a bronchial dilator, the same type of medicine that is used for asthma. However, it is best if your sister sees a doctor to get the proper treatment for her condition and her own inhaler.

Types of bronchitis

CAUSES	SYMPTOMS	ACTION
Acute bronchitis Bacteria or virus infection, often following a cold.	Head cold; runny nose; fever and chills; aching muscles.	Bed rest; aspirin; cough medicine; fluids; antibiotics; warm atmosphere.
Smoking.	Persistent cough: initially dry and racking, later loose and producing phlegm.	Stop smoking.
Chronic bronchitis Persistent irritation of the bronchial tubes; bacterial infection; irritation to damaged bronchial tubes and lungs.	Phlegm; cough; wheezing. Bronchitis without emphysema: shortness of breath during exercise; weight gain; bluish tinge to lips.	Stop smoking. Bronchial dilator drugs; physiotherapy of chest; postural drainage; yoga and breathing exercises; antibiotics.
Smoking; wet, cold climates; pollution; low resistance; fatigue.	Bronchitis with emphysema: shortness of breath; weight loss; barrel chest.	Severe cases may require hospitalization; oxygen, if necessary. Avoid bronchial irritants.

Monitoring lung function

The progress of lung damage in smokers can be accurately monitored by measuring the volume of air that can be expelled from the lungs in one second. This is called the forced expiratory volume (FEV), and the normal figure is about 1 gallon (3.8 l). If the airways are narrowed, this volume will be reduced. In healthy nonsmokers, the FEV begins to drop from about the age of 20 at an average rate of 0.67 to 1.35 fluid ounces (0.02 to 0.04 l) per year. In smokers with obstructive lung disease, the FEV drops two to three times faster than this. Treatment must therefore begin as soon as possible, starting with giving up smoking. Frequent, acute attacks worsen chronic bronchitis and make it harder to deal with. For these reasons preventive steps must also be taken to stem the progress of chronic bronchitis.

When people with mild to moderate airflow obstruction quit smoking, however, the rate of decline in FEV slows markedly and will eventually revert to that found in nonsmokers of the same age.

With smokers the rate of decline of lung function varies. A proportion of smokers with a persistent (chronic) cough and phlegm do not suffer breathlessness. In these cases lung function tests do not reveal any obstruction of airflow. However, most smokers with productive coughs later go on to develop significant narrowing of the lung airways.

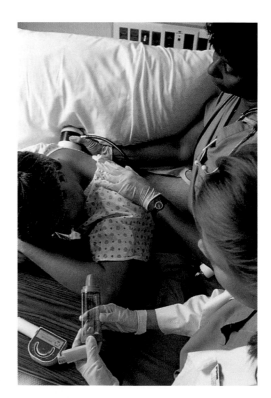

▲ *This physiotherapist is using a special electric device that emits vibrations to help loosen phlegm in the patient's lungs.*

See also: Asthma; Breathing; Coughing; Environmental hazards; Mucus; Phlegm; Physical therapy; Smoking; Wheezing

Brucellosis

Brucellosis is caused by various types of *Brucella* bacteria. It is an infection that primarily affects animals, although it can be transmitted to people by contact with infected animals, or via unpasteurized milk or dairy products.

Questions and Answers

How common is brucellosis in the United States?

It is a rare in the United States, even in cattle. In June 2000 there were only six infected herds, and 44 states were free of the disease. There are fewer than 100 human cases of brucellosis in the United States each year, most of which are ranchers, and the risk is decreasing: in 1946, there were 6,700 U.S. cases of brucellosis in humans, in 1997 there were only 98. Brucellosis in humans is rising worldwide, however, mainly because of infections acquired by travelers in countries where the disease is endemic.

Can brucellosis be passed on through food products?

Yes, although modern processing such as pasteurization of milk cuts the risk. Products such as cheeses made with unpasteurized milk do pose a small risk, particularly if imported from high-risk countries. Elderly and infirm people, and pregnant women should avoid such products. Properly cooked meat poses no threat of brucellosis.

How can I avoid brucellosis?

Unless you work very closely with animals, you are extremely unlikely to contract brucellosis. People who work with animals, and their physicians, should be aware of the risk and symptoms of brucellosis. Animal workers can reduce their chances of catching brucellosis through appropriate hygiene.

Even for those in the highest-risk professions, there is only a small chance of contracting brucellosis. The small risk from handling live animals is reduced by using protective gloves and disinfecting calving areas. Cattle abortions should be treated with particular care. Slaughterhouse workers should use protective gloves and clothing.

Brucellosis, also known as Malta fever or undulant fever, is a zoonosis—an infectious disease that people catch from animals. It is caused by bacteria in the genus *Brucella*. There are at least six species, two of which are of particular interest in the United States: *Brucella abortus* infects cattle; *B. suis* also infects cattle, but is more common in pigs and deer. *B. melitensis* infects goats and is the most contagious type for people, but it is unknown in the United States. Wild animals, camels, buffalo, and zoo animals also suffer from brucellosis. In the 1990s *Brucella* was discovered in seals in England. A form of brucellosis, *Brucella canis*, can also affect dogs.

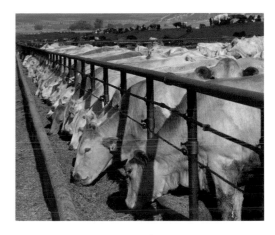

▲ *Farm animals such as cows contract the disease more often in developing countries.*

How do humans catch brucellosis?

There are two main methods of transmission to people: by eating untreated foodstuffs such as unpasteurized milk and by direct contact with infected animals. Infected animals shed bacteria through their milk. Using infected milk and milk products may cause the disease in humans. Discharges and afterbirth from an infected animal may also contain *Brucella* bacteria, and people may also be infected by inhaling airborne contamination from aborted animals. People such as ranchers and veterinarians, or others in direct contact with animals, are most at risk

Brucellosis affects the health and productivity of cattle. The commercial consequences for farmers whose livestock develop brucellosis are severe. Cattle lose weight and become infertile, and milk yields fall. The disease commonly causes spontaneous abortion in cattle. Some animals become lame. The disease spreads quickly within a herd because cows habitually lick each other and so pick up the bacteria from infected animals. Another risk of infection comes from sharing food and water. Brucellosis most commonly passes between herds when animals are moved or mixed before infection is detected within a herd. Another route for interherd infection is by contact with wild animals such as deer. These animals not only are susceptible to *Brucella* infection but may also share feeding areas with cattle and so pass on the disease.

National or state testing programs aim to discover brucellosis in livestock. Brucellosis infection was reduced hugely in North America and Europe during the 20th century. Infected animals are slaughtered, and restrictions on movement prevent interherd spread. Controls on the use of cattle products such as milk from infected animals protect human health. The disease remains prevalent in less developed areas, including countries such as Mexico. Cattle imported from countries where the disease remains common may bring infection with them. Imported milk or meat that has not been pasteurized or cooked may also expose people to infection.

In humans the incubation period can be just a day but is usually a week or two up to several months. Typical initial symptoms are fatigue and headaches. These progress to a fever similar to that in a bout of flu. Chills and sweats combine with aching limbs and joint and back pains. These symptoms are nonspecific, so diagnosis is difficult. The profession of the patient may give a clue: farmers, veterinarians, and others who work with animals are most likely to have contact with the disease. Infection rarely, if ever, passes between people. After antibiotic treatment most people recover within two to three weeks.

See also: Antibiotics; Bacteria; Diagnosis; Infection and infectious diseases

Bruises

Questions and Answers

My son bruised his shin really badly while playing football. Is it possible that he could have damaged the bone in some way?

Although the shinbone (tibia) is very near the surface of the skin, it is strong and does not fracture easily. Nevertheless, he should see a doctor if you are worried.

Is it true that children tend to bruise more easily than adults?

It often appears that children bruise more easily, but this is usually because of their nonstop activity, which makes them more prone to accidents. Children and adults who do seem to bruise more easily than other people should be checked by a doctor. The elderly do bruise more easily than younger people, because they lose the elasticity of their skin, and their capillaries (small blood vessels) become increasingly fragile.

I have noticed that my bruises take longer to fade than other people's. What is the reason?

Several factors could be adding to the delay. Your body's clearing mechanism may be slow in reaching the affected area, or the bruising may be extensive and so may take longer to clear anyway. Alternatively, if hematoma occurs, you may need medical help. Finally, there is a slight possibility that you may have a deficiency either of vitamin C or of blood platelets, which will slow down the clotting process. You should see your doctor.

My European neighbor said that her doctor once gave her pills to help her bruising. Is this normal?

In cases of severe bruising, some foreign doctors do prescribe pills, but this is not a common practice in the United States.

If a person is hit by a blunt or solid object, bruising usually occurs around the site of the blow. Severe bruising can lead to complications, but most bruises, although painful at first, will disappear within a few days.

A bruise, the result of damage to surface blood vessels, is a patch of dark or discolored skin. If the skin is unbroken, the bruise is known technically as a contusion. However, if it is more extensive, leading to the formation of a clotted lump of blood beneath the skin, it is called a hematoma.

Bruising can happen as the result of any sudden contact with a solid or blunt object. A single bump will result in a single contusion; the violent impact of a car accident, for example, could cause multiple bruises. If an accident occurs, causing bruising, the force may damage the small blood vessels—the capillaries—within the lining of the skin (see Capillaries). If an even greater force is applied, small veins may be broken (see Veins). This, in turn, could lead to the more massive form of bruising, a hematoma.

Symptoms

When a capillary breaks, blood oozes out—it is this internal bleeding that gives bruised skin its familiar dark-red color. Any bluish tinge is partly caused by a loss of oxygen in the red blood cells, although the thickness of the skin can also distort the color.

The puffiness of bruises is caused by the release of the serous fluid (white blood cells and platelets) in plasma (see Blood). The platelets initiate a process called coagulation or clotting. This limits the spread of the bruise and produces fibrin, a substance that helps plug the leaking blood vessels. A bruise takes between three and 14 days to clear, changing from reddish blue to greenish blue, and then yellow. These color changes arise from the body's efforts to reclaim the blood that has leaked into the tissues. It is this process that causes the bruise to slowly fade.

Treatment

Small bruises are best left to heal on their own. The only exception is a bruise under a toe- or fingernail, a condition known as subungeral hematoma. In this case medical advice should be sought because the end bone under the nail (the terminal phalanx) could be broken. The doctor may decide to release blood from under the nail, so relieving pain and reducing the risk of infection. When bruises occur with open wounds or lie over bony structures such as the skull and ribs, they may conceal a fracture. In the case of bruises to the face and scalp especially, it is always advisable to consult the doctor to rule out any underlying fracture or other damage.

For a contusion, first aid in the form of gentle compression to the injury, using either an ice pack or a cloth soaked in cold water, will limit the pain and swelling if applied quickly. Painkillers such as acetaminophen will ease discomfort and help reduce bruising. Aspirin, which is an anticlotting agent, should be avoided, since it can delay the healing process.

Larger bruises that result in hematoma should be seen by a doctor, who may decide to release the pressure of the blood by simple surgery. This will deprive bacteria in the damaged tissue of any nourishment. Failure to treat a boxer's hematoma can lead to a deformity called cauliflower ear.

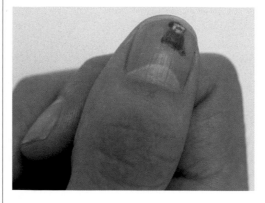

▲ *Sometimes, a bruised fingernail may cover a small broken bone.*

See also: **Aspirin and analgesics; Bacteria; Black eye; Fractures; Infection and infectious diseases; Painkillers; Plasma; Swellings; Vitamin C; Wounds**

Bunions

Wearing poorly made and badly shaped shoes can result in bunions—an unsightly and painful foot deformity that may require surgery. Prevention simply involves a little care in choosing comfortable shoes that fit well.

Bunions can begin at any age, especially if your child has broad feet. Avoid passing on shoes from one child to another, because the inside of each shoe is shaped to the original wearer's foot. No two feet are exactly alike, even within a family. When children are growing quickly, they are especially at risk.

I have very bad bunions. Is my young son likely to inherit them?

This depends whether your bunions are caused by tight shoes or an inherited predisposition. Your condition is probably due to a little of both. Your son will likely inherit your tendency, but boys' shoes tend to be wider, so he should not develop bunions.

I thought I had a bad bunion, but my doctor tells me it is gout. What is the difference?

Gout is a type of arthritis that commonly affects the big toe joint. The painful, red swelling that results may resemble a bunion, but gout comes on suddenly whereas a bunion develops much more slowly. However, an infected bunion could resemble gout, so if there is sudden pain when your foot is at rest, you should consult your doctor.

My teenage daughter likes to buy outrageous shoes with high heels and pointed toes. How can I stop her from ruining her feet?

Show her photos of the feet of women who wore such shoes, and who now must see a podiatrist. Your daughter and some of her more sensible friends might make a project of finding stylish but safer alternatives.

A bunion, which arises as a result of pressure, is an abnormal enlargement at the joint between the foot and the beginning of the big toe. All joints are surrounded by a capsule of fibrous tissue. There may also be a bag of fluid, called a bursa, which cushions the movements of the various parts of the joint (see Bursitis). When the big toe joint becomes swollen and inflamed, more fluid collects there and the ends of the bones may actually enlarge. Then, instead of lying in a straight line, the joint is forced outward at an angle. This puts pressure on the tissues between the bones and the shoe, resulting in the formation of a bunion. The overlying skin may also become thickened and inflamed. Matters are made worse by the fact that all this happens just where most shoes rub.

How bunions develop

Distortion of the big toe joint is usually caused by wearing shoes that are too tight for the toes. Traditionally, women's shoes are made narrower at the front than men's, although the anatomy of male and female feet is the same, so women tend to develop bunions more often than men.

The problem is increased because women's shoes have higher heels. These force the foot deep into the tight front of the shoe and put maximum pressure on the side of the big toe. If this sideways pressure continues day after day, the big toe joint is pushed out of place and becomes deformed, leading to a condition called hallux valgus. The big toe begins to point across the other toes, and the foot bone leading to the big toe begins to point outward. Once this condition becomes established, any further pressure from shoes will fall almost entirely on the big toe joint and will cause a bunion. At the other side of the foot a similar deformity can arise, causing a small bunion to form at the little toe joint.

Some people are born with a tendency to develop hallux valgus and are therefore more likely to develop bunions. This may be because they have feet that are unusually broad in front, so that off-the-rack shoes never fit properly. More rarely, a person may be born with the foot bone leading to the big toe abnormally developed and already pointing outward.

Whatever the cause, this deformity, once started, will tend to become worse and will not repair itself, even if no shoes at all are worn. This is because the tendons running to the toe bones become displaced. Instead of lying directly over the joint, they pull across to the inside. Then, every time the muscles contract to flex or extend the big toe—as happens at every step during walking—the pull of the tendons makes the condition worse.

Prevention and treatment

Some of the modern-day shoe manufacturers have responded to public concerns about foot

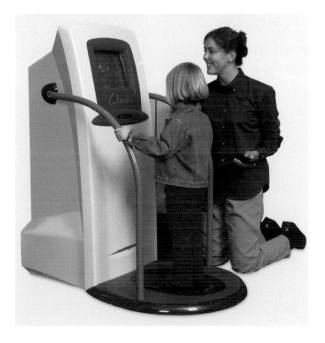

▶ *If children have their feet properly measured and their parents buy them well-fitted shoes, they should avoid developing bunions.*

deformities caused by poor-fitting fashion shoes. As a result, some wider shoes with lower heels are now available in attractive styles. Shoes with very high heels and pointed toes that are worn regularly are bound to lead to problems, even in those who have narrow feet. Anyone who feels pain or notices redness of the skin on the outside of the big toe should immediately throw out their shoes.

To see just how much room their feet take up, people should stand barefoot on a tape measure and compare the width of their toes with that allowed by their shoes. There is always a difference, and this difference represents the pressure that is being taken by their toes.

Owing to the taut, bowstring effect on the tendons, treatment options for bunions tend to be unsatisfactory. Wide-toed shoes are essential. A special pad may be worn between the big and index toes to try to correct the alignment of the big toe and to reduce pressure on the bunion. In the end, many women feel they have no alternative but to get an operation. Prevention is better than cure, so it is better to keep the problem from arising in the first place.

Complications

On its own a bunion is not a serious condition. Occasionally, however, it can become infected and will then require immediate treatment. This complication may be caused by attempting to pare down the thickened skin as if it were a corn—this should never be done (see Corns).

HOW BUNIONS ARE CAUSED

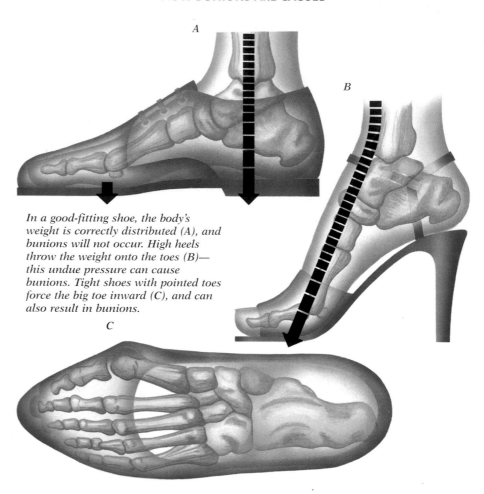

In a good-fitting shoe, the body's weight is correctly distributed (A), and bunions will not occur. High heels throw the weight onto the toes (B)— this undue pressure can cause bunions. Tight shoes with pointed toes force the big toe inward (C), and can also result in bunions.

Nor should a blister that may have formed over a bunion be opened. Once the skin is broken, infection can quickly spread to the fluid of the bunion and then to the big toe joint. The joint will become even more swollen, red, and painful, and eventually pus may be discharged from it.

Treatment with antibiotics is then urgent to prevent any further spread of the infection and avoid septic destruction of the joint. If the sufferer is also run-down, the infection may take a long time to clear up (see Blisters; Infection and Infectious Diseases). Another complication can be that, as a long-term result of hallus valgus, the abnormal alignment of the big toe joint causes excessive wear and tear and, consequently, arthritis (see Joints). In addition, if the pain of a bunion has made a person walk in an abnormal way to compensate for the pain, there is a possibility that arthritis could also develop in other joints.

Surgery

Bunions can be unsightly, but surgeons are reluctant to operate on them if the only purpose is cosmetic. Merely cutting out the bunion is never sufficient, as the trouble will only recur. Rather, a full operation must be performed to correct the deformity, one that actually removes the offending joint by cutting away the bone. Eventually, the bone that has been cut out is replaced by strong bands of fibrous tissue that grow in its place. This tissue allows some degree of movement, but it will never be able to function like a joint.

After the operation, it will take some time before the patient can walk again without it being painful. For about three months wearing any type of shoe will hurt, and most people do not feel that they have received any benefit from the operation until about six months have elapsed. The patient is usually advised to wear orthopedic shoes, at least during the recovery period.

Footnotes
Do not start your children wearing shoes too early—let them go barefoot wherever it is safe to do so.
Discard shoes as soon as they are too small—even when they are great favorites.
Have your child's feet measured regularly, every two months.
Discourage teenage girls from wearing stiletto heels— especially if there is a tendency toward bunions in the family.

See also: Antibiotics; Bones; Cosmetic surgery; Feet; Muscles; Pain; Posture; Surgery; Swellings; Tendons

Burn center

Questions and Answers

How are new technologies affecting the care of burn patients?

Improvements include the use of antimicrobial dressings such as Acticoat7 to reduce the risk of infection; the use of ultrasound to assess the severity of the wound, since ultrasound avoids bodily contact that would cause the patient more pain; and the use of virtual reality to manage pain.

A key development is the creation of artificial skins, such as Integra TM, through tissue engineering. Bioengineered skin avoids the repeated surgery and complications associated with skin replacements from other sources, which the patient might reject.

What can be done to improve the quality of life for survivors?

As survival rates improve, the focus is on the survivors' quality of life. Accredited burn centers are required to provide suitable aftercare to ensure that their patients regain as much body function as possible and get counseling for emotional and psychological problems. Studies show that children's quality of life, in particular, depends less on the extent of their disability than on the support of their family and family counselors. Survivors' quality of life may be improved ' by new techniques that minimize permanent scarring, including dermabrasion, laser surgery, micropigmentation, and skin expansion. Burn support centers, such as the Foundation for Burns and Trauma, run holiday camps, advice centers, and Websites.

What is the long-term outlook for burn centers?

After 11 September 2001, under bioterrorism legislation approved in June 2002, burn centers in the United States received an extra $1.6 billion funding.

Burn care is evolving, and technological advances are expected to shorten recovery times and reduce risks for patients. Special dressings and artificial skin, which are used in burn centers, have improved the care of burn victims.

A burn center is a specialized care facility dedicated to the treatment and rehabilitation of burn patients. There are around 200 burn centers in the United States, where more than two million burn injuries are reported a year. Of these two million patients, between 8,000 and 12,000 will die and up to one million will be left with a permanent disability. Advances at burn centers are the main reason why far fewer people are likely to die from burn injuries today than 20 years ago, and advances have also made it possible for many more burn patients to lead independent lives after being discharged from the hospital.

Burns are among the most traumatic of all injuries and put a unique stress on the human body (see Burns). The skin is the body's largest organ, and severe burns compromise the skin's four main functions: preventing the loss of body fluids, protecting against infection, regulating body temperature, and providing sensory contact (see Skin and Skin Diseases). Severe burns can even lead to major organ failure. The severity of a burn injury is classified depending on its depth. First-degree burns damage the epidermis or outer layer of skin. Second-degree burns damage the epidermis and part of the dermis, the inner layer of skin. Third-degree burns damage dermis and epidermis, and possibly bones, nerves, and tendons as well. Most second-degree and all third-degree burns require a stay in the hospital, roughly at least a day for each percent of the body burned. Many patients visit a burn center as outpatients for up to a year after an injury.

In addition to the physical and physiological impact of being severely burned, a burn patient often suffers lasting emotional and psychological effects. Caring for a burn patient requires a comprehensive, multidisciplinary approach that takes into account all aspects of a patient's recovery, from controlling pain and managing the wound to reintegrating the patient into life as fully as possible. Thus, burn center staff includes surgeons, cardiac specialists, plastic and reconstructive surgeons, burn nurses, anesthetists, respiratory therapists, pharmacy consultants,

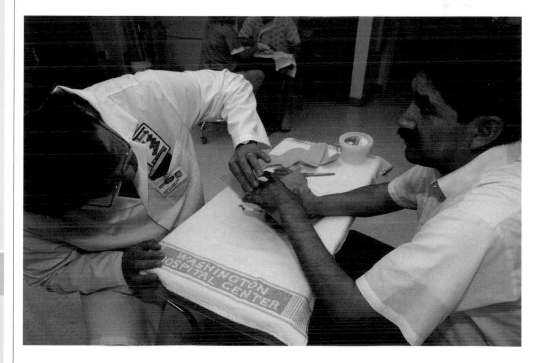

▲ *A firefighter receives specialized treatment for his burned hand in the burn unit at Washington Hospital Center.*

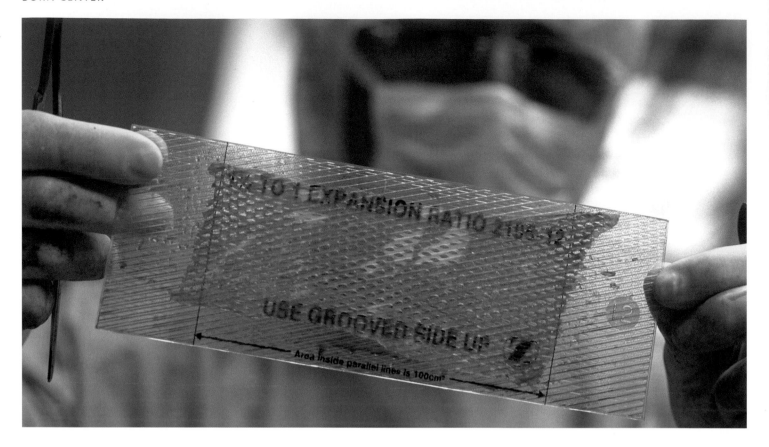

▲ *A strip of skin is worked and prepared for transplant at a specialist burn center at Cochin hospital.*

occupational therapists, social workers, psychiatrists, chaplains, and dieticians, among others. Although burn injuries last a lifetime, these specialists can alleviate their effects through rehabilitation programs that promote the patient's overall health.

Burn centers are often attached to hospital trauma centers, with which they may share facilities. Burn centers in the United States vary considerably in size—the largest is the William Randolph Hearst Burn Center in New York, which has 48 beds and treats up to 1,000 inpatients and 4,000 outpatients annually. In the early stages of their treatment, burn patients make regular visits to the tank room, where they lie on a stainless steel table and are sprayed with water by hoses hanging from the ceiling. Here, as in the hydrotherapy room where patients bathe, water removes the damaged skin and leaves the wound exposed.

Burn patients have difficulty regulating their body temperature, and all operating theaters and rooms have heating lamps. Leading burn centers, such as the William Randolph Hearst Burn Center, may have hyperbaric oxygen chambers where the patient is exposed to an oxygenated atmosphere at a pressure much higher than atmospheric pressure to treat wounds that will not heal and skin grafts. Rehabilitation rooms and exercise facilities are also found at a burn center, as are skin banks where donor skin is kept for grafts.

Treatment and rehabilitation

The burn patient's journey to recovery is long and complex, involving often painful treatments and close monitoring of all aspects of his or her health. On arrival at a burn center, the patient is assessed, and steps are taken to prevent fluid loss and infection. Once the patient is stabilized, pain is managed by specialist anesthetists, and wounds are cleaned and covered by burn nurses, who change the dressings twice a day. Physical and occupational therapists assist patients with stretching exercises and pressure garments that help to prevent tightening of the scar. The therapists help position patients to avoid contractures and help patients maintain and increase their range of motion. Burn patients have particular nutritional needs, and dieticians devise high-protein, high-carbohydrate diets to promote skin regrowth and overall health. Social workers assist with other matters arising from an injury, such as loss of income, legal assistance, or arranging home education for children. Severe burns can cause disabilities, such as amputation, disfigurement, or loss of bodily function, which have emotional effects on the patient and his or her family. Psychiatrists, counselors, and chaplains discuss the patient's concerns and put him or her in touch with burn survivors' groups. This intervention continues as part of a rehabilitation program after the patient returns home.

Surgical treatments

One priority in a burn patient's recovery is replacing burned skin to restore the body's protective barrier against infection. Depending on the size of the burned area, artificial or donor skin may be grafted onto damaged skin, or the patient's own skin cells may be used to culture new skin for grafts (see Grafting). Burn patients may have to undergo other surgical procedures to lessen scarring, including dermabrasion, which involves shaving or scraping off the top layers of skin. Many such developments have arisen from research by scientists at burn centers.

See also: **Counseling; Infection and infectious diseases; Physical therapy; Wounds**

Burns

Questions and Answers

My mother always believed in putting butter or olive oil on a burn she got while cooking. Is either any good as a burn dressing?

No. Both oil and butter act as food for bacteria, which can develop and increase the risk of infecting the burn. For the same reason, you should never use ointments on burns; use clean, dry dressings on their own instead.

How do I know when a burn is serious enough that I should call a doctor or go to a hospital?

If in any doubt, seek medical help immediately, particularly for burns on the face or genitals, over a joint, or in the mouth or throat; burns larger than 3 sq. in. (20 cm²); burns that are wet and oozing; burns that continue to hurt in spite of first aid; burns caused by electricity; and burns in someone very young or old.

I read that it is not a good idea to drive a burn victim to the hospital yourself. Wouldn't this save time?

Not if you were stopped by the police on the way—remember, you do not have the same priority in traffic as an ambulance. Besides, your patient may need to be lying down and could vomit or lose consciousness as you drive, when you couldn't do anything to help.

Should I see a doctor if I get sunburned on vacation?

Yes, if the sunburn is severe or is combined with sunstroke. You should take care to get used to the sun gradually if you are fair-skinned or unused to strong sunlight. You can even get sunburned on ice and snow on a mountaintop, owing to the reflected ultraviolet radiation from the sun. Also, if you are on a beach, the sun is more intense near the sea and sand than elsewhere.

The best way to deal with burns is to take all the necessary precautions to prevent them. However, if an accident does happen, knowing what to do could mean the difference between life and death.

Every day, countless people die from or are severely injured by burns. Although it is generally assumed that the main cause is fire, burns can also result from touching hot objects or be caused by scalding, harsh friction, electric shock, or accidental contact with corrosive chemicals. The injury can be even greater if the victims are either very young or old. Very old people have the poorest chance of recovery from severe burns, but children are also vulnerable, especially toddlers who do not understand the dangers involved in playing with fire.

Lesser burns
A burn is classified medically according to the depth that it reaches in the skin. There are three types: these are usually referred to as first-, second-, and third-degree burns. In the first group, also called superficial partial-thickness burns, the epidermis (outer layer) of the skin is destroyed and the dermis (thicker, underlying tissues) may also be affected. But the hair follicles, sweat glands, and basic structure remain to form a basis for the growth of healthy new skin (see Skin and Skin Diseases). The minor burns that happen in the kitchen or from sunburn fall into this category. The pain will stop within a few days, and the skin will soon recover. Sometimes a blister is formed; this protects the underlying wound from infection and should not be pricked. All the affected part needs is to be covered with a clean, dry dressing and allowed to heal (see Blisters).

More serious burns
In the second group—deep partial-thickness burns—all but the deepest cells, hair follicles, and glands are destroyed. With this type of burn, healing is slow, and the new skin that is produced is likely to be rough and not as elastic as before.

The most serious type of burn is classified as a third-degree burn. Here the whole thickness burns, completely destroying the cellular structure of the skin; there is nothing from which the new skin can reform, unless it is at the very edges of the burn. In this event healing is extremely

SKIN DEPTHS OF FIRST-, SECOND-, AND THIRD-DEGREE BURNS

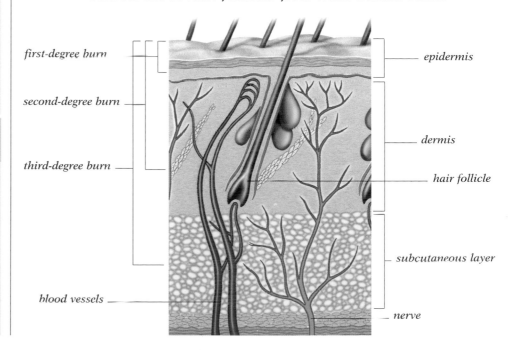

first-degree burn

second-degree burn

third-degree burn

blood vessels

epidermis

dermis

hair follicle

subcutaneous layer

nerve

303

TREATING BURNS

▼ *The first treatment for every burn is to cool it off. For scalds, remove any clothing that has become hot from boiling fluid, fat, or steam. However, if the clothing has already cooled, do not remove it.*

▼ *A chemical burn can be very nasty, so quickly remove any soaked clothing without touching the chemical yourself. Immediately wash away the chemical by flooding the area with water for at least ten minutes.*

▼ *An electrical burn requires fast action. Do not touch the victim until you have switched off the current. If this is impossible, call the power company or 911 immediately. Do not touch anything in contact with a downed wire.*

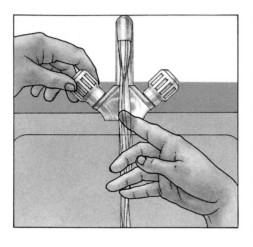

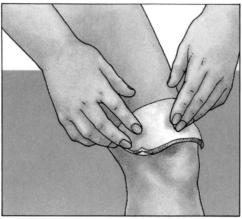

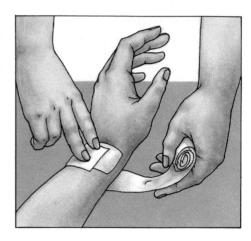

Always begin by cooling the burn. Heat from a burn can cause major damage that penetrates deep into the body. Applying cold water helps reduce this effect. A small part, like a fingertip or wrist, can be held under a running tap; a larger area should be plunged into a bucket or sink full of cold water.

Areas like the face or chest that cannot be kept under water should be covered by a thick cloth soaked in cold water for at least ten minutes. This quickly relieves pain and reduces the formation of blisters. If the cloth gets warm and dry, renew cold water and reapply. If much pain persists, repeat the procedure.

A large burn or a burn on the face should be covered with a nonfluffy dry dressing after cooling. Use the inside of a sterile surgical dressing or a clean handkerchief, handling it as little as possible. Do not apply lotion or ointment, and avoid touching the burn. Cover with more folded padding, and bandage loosely.

slow and uncertain. The whole area is more or less free of pain because the nerve endings have been destroyed. But pain cannot be entirely absent, for at the edges of the burn there are likely to be some areas where nerve endings remain.

The loss of plasma (the colorless, liquid part of the blood) is one of the major problems with severe burns. Burns can form blisters that are filled with plasma which oozes out from the damaged blood vessels in the surrounding area (see Blood). The blood cells are left behind. From this point of view, the area covered by a burn is more significant than the depth. Plasma, although it is colorless and without its cells, is still blood fluid, and a dramatic drop in its volume contributes to the condition known as shock. To make matters worse, the remaining blood in the body is now thicker, since its cells are concentrated in a smaller amount of plasma—this increases the difficulties of the heart, which may already be under stress.

Another problem is that a surface coating of plasma on the wound makes infection by bacteria much more likely. A great deal of protein is also lost, together with the plasma.

Hospital treatment

Deep and extensive burns require hospital treatment. Relief of pain is, of course, important, but the primary concern is to combat shock.

The percentage of skin area that has been burned is also an important factor in deciding what treatment is to be given—for example, the back or front of the trunk represents 18 percent of the whole surface of the body, while a hand represents 1 percent.

A transfusion is likely to be needed when the burned area represents more than 15 percent of the total skin surface in an adult or more than 10 percent in a child. The fluid is generally plasma, but sometimes whole blood is included to replace red blood cells that have been destroyed (see Plasma). Also, the patient's general condition must be closely watched, as the burned area will have lost much of its natural defense against bacteria. Not only does infection delay healing; it also increases the risk of disfigurement from scarring, and scars may contract and interfere with the movement of any joint they overlie. Antibiotics will be prescribed to combat any infection and thereby help the healing process.

A partial-thickness burn is generally allowed to heal spontaneously, either by being left exposed or by being covered with a dressing. Healing may take between two and three months.

A full-thickness burn will not mend in this way, because the regenerating tissue has been destroyed. The dead material eventually separates off as dark, hard slough, leaving a raw area below. Frequently, it has to be helped off gently by doctors and nurses, and a skin graft will be necessary to close up the wound.

When a skin graft is performed, small pieces of skin are removed from another part of the patient's body (usually from a place that is ordinarily covered by clothing). This healthy skin is implanted into the burned area and gradually grows to reform a new skin surface (see Grafting). Skin grafting demands several months of skillful care; and it is especially important to ensure that the grafted skin does not contract, since contracting can affect the joint below.

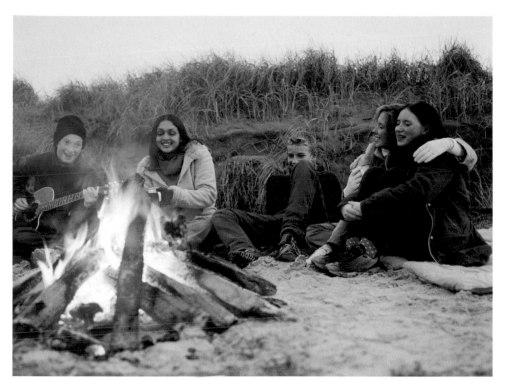

▲ *People often congregate around a campfire to keep warm, but care should be taken. If a person is standing too close to the flames, any loose clothing can catch fire. In such cases, douse the flames with water or smother them with a heavy material.*

Preventing fires and burns

Smoking: Stub out cigarettes thoroughly in ashtray. Do not throw cigarette stubs into a wastepaper basket. Do not smoke in bed or near inflammable material—for instance, in a garage.

Cooking: Light match before turning on gas tap. Never hang cloths over oven. Fill deep fryer no more than halfway and watch constantly; have large metal lid handy to smother flames in case of fire, and keep fire blanket by cooker for same purpose. Never put a hand in front of steam from kettle.

Heating: Have sturdy fireguards. Sweep chimneys regularly. Do not use paraffin or gasoline to light fires. Keep rugs away from fireplace. Ban toys from mantelpiece, and never place mirror on wall above fire. Be sure oil heaters are firmly based, and don't fill or carry them when they are lit.

Clothes: Beware of light cotton fabrics. Buy flameproof nightwear for children and old people.

Wiring: Replace frayed electric wires, loose connections, and trailing leads. Fit correct fuses. Switch off to disconnect apparatus not in use; always pull out plug. Do not connect heaters or irons to lamp sockets.

General planning: Keep a fire extinguisher handy. Clear papers and rags from attic or under stairs.

Victims of severe burns may need a high-calorie diet rich in protein and vitamins, with extra iron to replace what has been lost in the plasma. Other organs, located far away from the burn, such as the liver, stomach, intestines, gallbladder, and kidney, may also have been damaged. This is because shock following the burn reduces blood supply to vital organs, causing damage that will not appear immediately. These organs are kept under surveillance while the patient is in the hospital. Physiotherapy will be given as soon as possible to maintain movement and the health and fitness of undamaged limbs (see Physical Therapy).

What to do in case of fire

If someone is trapped by a fire, a rescuer should cover his or her nose and mouth with a wet cloth. It is better to reach the victim by crawling on the floor, where smoke is less dense, and guide or pull the victim out. If the victim is choked by hot fumes, artificial respiration should be given. Victims may panic and run around beating at their clothes—actions that are likely to fan the flames. The rescuer should try to stop this by getting the victim on the floor, with the burning area uppermost to allow flames to rise away from the body. Flames should be extinguished with water if possible; or, the flames can be smothered with thick material such as a rug, heavy towel, or coat. This should be thrown toward the victim's feet, directing the flames away from the face. Air can be excluded by pressing down gently but any hot, smoldering cloth should not be pressed against the victim's skin. The cloth should be pulled away, but without tearing away any material sticking to the skin. The victim must not be rolled; this would expose different areas to the flames.

Other forms of treatment

With a bad burn, the risk of shock is high. Shock is treated by lying the victim down, loosening any tight clothing, and covering him or her lightly. The victim can be given a cupful of water, to be sipped every 15 minutes. Rescuers should aim to be reassuring and calm, but they should send for an ambulance immediately (see Shock). Any charred but cold material sticking to the skin should be left in place, but jewelry, such as a ring, bracelet, or necklace, that could constrict the burned area (which may swell) may be removed. A blister must be left alone and nothing but cold water applied to it. If no surgical dressings are handy, a clean handkerchief or towel may be used. For maximum hygiene, the dressing should be handled by one corner and the inside surface used on the burn, followed by a padding of more folded material (another clean handkerchief or small towel) and secured with an improvised bandage, such as a necktie or panty hose. If the face is burned, holes can be cut in the dressing to let the patient see. However, badly swollen eyelids may keep the eyes closed. The victim must be moved only to raise a burned limb; this helps to reduce swelling. The victim should be constantly reassured.

See also: **Artificial respiration; Blood transfusion; Plasma; Protein; Resuscitation; Scars**

Burping

Questions and Answers

My husband and his family seem to have a burping problem. Can this run in families?

Yes. If it is acceptable behavior in his family to burp, then family members will be unlikely to suppress the habit. However, it should be possible to persuade your husband to control his burping if you want him to conform to the social norm. It may be simply a matter of reviewing his eating and drinking.

My brother is always burping and claims he cannot help it. Why is he doing this?

The most likely cause is that he is swallowing air, although your brother may be unaware of this. If he has no other gastric symptoms, it is most unlikely that this is a medical problem.

My baby cries a lot after he has been fed. I spend ages trying to burp him, but nothing happens. Am I doing anything wrong?

No. He's probably not bringing up gas because he has not swallowed much air. It does not sound as if gas is the problem here.

Can a good, loud burp show appreciation of a good meal?

In American society, a burp is considered antisocial. In some countries where eating is considered a pleasure of life, and the stomach distension of a good meal can be relieved by burping, it can be seen as a compliment.

Do men burp more than women?

No—both sexes have an equal tendency to burp. However, men tend to overindulge more in food and beer, both of which cause an excess of gas.

Burping, or bringing up gas, is a normal reflex action in babies after a meal. Adults, too, may suffer from excessive gas in the stomach, but they can learn to control the response—if they so choose.

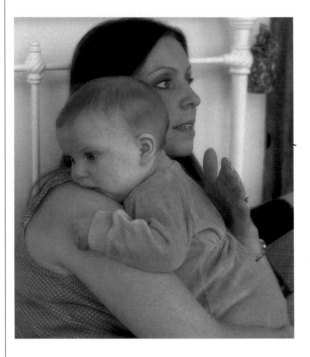

◀ *Helping a baby to bring up gas is best done by placing the child on a shoulder and firmly patting his or her back.*

Burping (belching) is the involuntary reflex (backward flow) of gas from the stomach and out of the mouth. With every mouthful of food that a person swallows, some air is also taken down into their stomach. Babies swallow a lot of air as they suck their milk—the actual amount varies with how well and how hard the baby sucks and how much milk is available from the breast or bottle.

Adults, too, often swallow excessive amounts of air, and this results in uncontrollable burps. Carbonated (fizzy) drinks contain dissolved gas, which is quickly released in the stomach. This can also cause burping, as can air swallowed to cool the taste of very hot food or to hide the taste of unpleasant food. People who eat too quickly and swallow a lot of air are often prone to burping and sharp stomach pain (see Indigestion).

How it happens

Once in the stomach, air can escape in two directions. First, it can pass on with the food into the small intestine. This passage is closed immediately after a meal to ensure that food is adequately digested in the stomach before being allowed to progress down to the gut. Alternatively, the air can return back up the esophagus (the tube that extends from the throat to the stomach) to the mouth. Then, any excessive buildup of gas will put pressure on the valve at the stomach entrance, which is also closed to prevent food from being regurgitated (vomited).

As the stomach churns away, digesting the food, the pressure of the air may get to be too much for the stomach valve. A burst of gas is released up the esophagus without warning.

Prevention

Burping is a natural phenomenon. Children are usually taught to control their burps, since the habit is considered antisocial in most cultures. Eating more slowly and not swallowing too much air along with hot or spicy food will prevent excessive burping.

In babies up to six months old, burping may cause concern. After being fed, babies should not be put directly to bed, because the air in their stomach could lead to pain and discomfort. Cuddling will be appreciated, during which babies may burp a little naturally. Parents will often use traditional methods of bringing up gas if a baby appears uncomfortable, such as placing the baby over a shoulder and patting his or her back gently but firmly. Preparations designed to help eliminate gas, often containing an herb such as fennel, may help in some cases.

See also: **Breast-feeding; Breathing; Digestive system; Esophagus; Flatulence; Pain; Reflexes; Stomach**

Bursitis

Now known to be a more complex process than was formerly understood, bursitis causes inflammation around joints and other bones. It includes the disorder called the impingement syndrome and is common in athletes.

A bursa is a protective fluid-filled pouch formed in soft tissue, usually overlying a bone or joint. Bursitis is the inflammation of one of these sacs. It is a common, and occasionally painful, condition requiring prompt treatment to stop the inflammation from becoming acute or chronic.

There are two types of bursa. The most common type, known as anatomical bursas, occur on specific sites where tendons cross bones or joints (see Tendons). There are 15 such bursas around the knee joint alone. People are usually unaware of these until they enlarge and bursitis develops. The second type of bursa is one that arises purely as a result of repeated friction or injury to soft tissue overlying a bony surface. These are known as adventitious bursas. They may develop, for example, over the pelvic bone in the buttock from sitting on a hard seat for several hours a day.

Bursas act as shock absorbers and pressure pads, reducing friction where tendons or ligaments move over bones (see Ligaments). Only when the bursa becomes chronically enlarged or acutely inflamed will bursitis develop. Prepatellar bursa, a condition that used to be called housemaid's knee—which develops in the largest bursa above the knee, anatomically known as the suprapatellar bursa—is caused by repeated pressure to the knee. Any friction or injury causes the bursa to secrete fluid, resulting in the swelling.

Causes

The causes of bursitis are not always clear. Although it can affect both children and adults, some people are more liable to develop the condition than others. When friction causes a bursa to develop, the condition may be due to the way certain occupations or activities are carried out. Bursitis of the elbow, for instance, is common among students who lean on desks and miners who crawl along tunnels. Porters sometimes develop bursitis at the neck from the pressure caused by carrying heavy boxes or baskets, as do construction workers from balancing loads of bricks. Weavers, who sit for long periods on hard loom seats, can develop bursitis on the buttocks; gardeners, who work from a kneeling position, are more likely to develop bursitis on the knees.

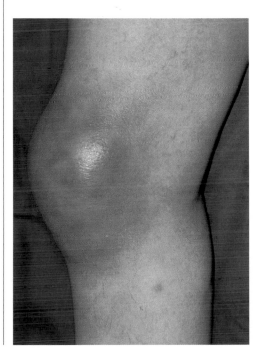

However, the effects of rubbing or friction are not the only explanation. In rarer cases bursitis can be caused by bacterial inflammation in the bursa or in a connecting joint. Tuberculosis was a common cause in the past. In some cases of rheumatoid arthritis, the bursa around a joint becomes inflamed (see Rheumatoid Arthritis), and in rare cases gout may develop in a bursa (see Gout). In bursitis of the elbow, which is common in older men, a cause is rarely identified at all, yet within a matter of hours a swelling the size of a chicken's egg can appear.

Symptoms

In cases of acute bursitis, a swelling appears over the joint or bone. The swollen area is painful, is tender to touch, and may feel hot

◄ *Formerly known as housemaid's knee, a prepatellar bursa can easily be prevented by simple measures.*

A COMMON SITE OF BURSITIS

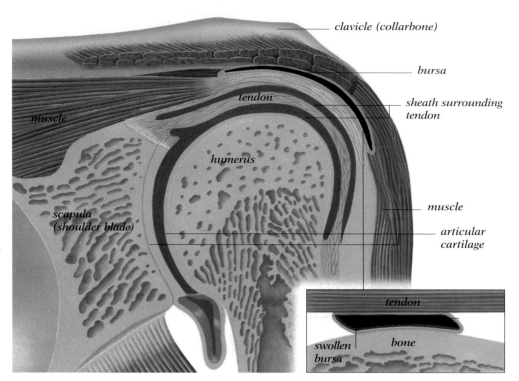

clavicle (collarbone)

bursa

sheath surrounding
tendon

tendon

muscle

humerus

muscle

scapula
(shoulder blade)

articular
cartilage

tendon

bone

swollen
bursa

◀ *In a normal shoulder (left), the bursa stops the tendon from rubbing on the shoulder joint. If undue pressure is put on a shoulder, the bursa will become inflamed and sore (insert). This inflammation can be avoided by padding the area.*

Impingement syndrome

"Impingement syndrome" is a term for a group of conditions affecting various parts of the body, particularly the shoulder, that were formerly described by other terms, including bursitis. These conditions are most commonly seen in people who practice sports that involve throwing and swimming. These activities require an abnormally frequent impingement, or striking, of one internal structure on another. This is especially the case when the arm is rotated outward and moved away from the body, and when it is moved repetitively in and above the horizontal plane.

Repetitive overhead use of the arm causes the tendons of the rotator cuff to rub against the shoulder blade and its ligaments. The rotator cuff consists of the tendons of four adjacent muscles, blended with the capsule of the joint.

One of these muscles, the supraspinatus, becomes inflamed and weakened by repetitive use. When this happens, the rotator cuff is no longer able to depress the head of the upper arm bone (the humerus) into its shallow socket, and the more powerful deltoid (shoulder-pad) muscle causes the head of the humerus to ride up, altering the way the joint works and making the situation worse. Considerable inflammation of tendons and bursas results, and inflamed tissue causes further impingement and damage.

Stages of the syndrome

The syndrome can be divided into three stages. The first resembles simple bursitis, with inflammation and swelling from fluid production (edema) of the rotator cuff. The bursa lying under the shoulder blade (the subachromial bursa) often becomes greatly swollen. In the second stage, pressure effects lead to an inadequate blood supply to the rotator cuff, and progressive degeneration and scarring result. The third stage involves a partial or complete tear.

Treatment

The treatment for acute bursitis should be supervised by a doctor, in case the cause is bacterial infection or another rare condition. If the cause is unknown, or if the bursitis is due to rubbing, friction, or excess use, then resting the affected joint or area, with only passive exercise for the surrounding muscles, is the cure.

If the condition is painful, painkillers may be necessary. Anti-inflammatory drugs, such as those used to treat arthritis, may reduce the amount of fluid secreted by the cells lining the bursa. Antibiotics are necessary only if there is also a bacterial infection present (see Infection and Infectious Diseases).

and appear red. Movement is often very painful. The fluid in acute bursitis is produced by the cells that line the wall of the sac. The cells produce a straw-colored fluid, often tinged with blood, as inflammation causes small blood vessels to leak. Where there is bacterial infection, this fluid becomes filled with bacteria and white blood cells to form pus, which may discharge (see Pus). Chronic bursitis is caused by repeated attacks of acute bursitis or repeated injury causing swelling of a bursa. Painful or even painless swelling may follow exercise or injury.

Bursitis is hardly ever dangerous. Spread of bacteria, septicemia (blood poisoning), and spread of tuberculosis are rarely seen in these days of antibiotics. Untreated gout or rheumatoid arthritis may cause harmful inflammation elsewhere in the body, and chronic, unattended bursitis will eventually lead to wasting of the surrounding muscles, which in turn may weaken the joint.

Occupational hazards

Traditionally, most causes of bursitis in Western societies were occupation-related. Health and safety regulations now, to a large extent, control the damage that may be done to workers by pressure effects of this kind. The replacement of unskilled labor by machinery has also greatly reduced the incidence of most early types of bursitis.

These former occupational cases have now been replaced by a rising incidence of sports-related conditions that are essentially self-inflicted. Sports used to be played largely for the pleasure of playing, rather than for the satisfaction of winning. Today, competitive pressures drive people, especially professional athletes, to make unprecedented demands on their bodies. Advances in orthopedics and sports medicine have shown that some of the conditions formerly described as bursitis actually involve far more complex causes than the production of excess fluid in bursas as a result of repeated pressure (see Sports Injury).

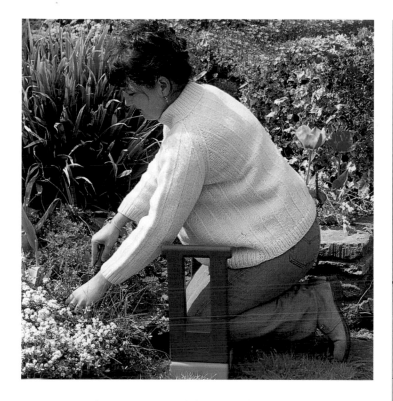

▲ *Eager gardeners can avoid the risk of bursitis by using a special kneeling pad for tasks such as weeding.*

How to avoid bursitis

PREPATELLAR BURSITIS

Avoid kneeling for any length of time when doing housework.

Never shuffle on your knees when you are working in a kneeling position.

If you have been kneeling for a length of time and your knees feel sore afterward, apply an elastic bandage to knees.

Use rubber kneeling pads for domestic work or gardening—this spreads the pressure over a larger area and is softer on the knees.

OTHER FORMS OF BURSITIS

Pad any area that is going to be subjected to pressure, for example, from a baby carrier, knapsack, trash can, or heavy basket. Plastic foam can be useful for padding.

Avoid tight, poor-fitting shoes, especially if you have bunions.

Wear thick clothing when carrying heavy objects. If leaning on one elbow is unavoidable when you are carrying out a task, make a habit of using elbow pads.

Athletes who practice sports involving throwing and swimming should be sure to report any persistent shoulder pain to a sports physician or physiotherapist.

In addition to resting the affected joint, a cold compress or ice pack may help reduce the inflammation. Cool a plastic bag filled with glycerin or crushed ice in the refrigerator. Then mold the cold bag to the contours of the skin, checking that it is not so cold as to irritate the affected area. Bandage lightly with a stretch bandage. Keep this on for half an hour. If this treatment provides relief, repeat as often as possible, up to once every four hours, until the condition improves.

If the condition does not improve within two or three days, the doctor may aspirate (drain) the bursa, using a hypodermic needle. First a local anesthetic is applied; then the needle is inserted deep into the bursa. Some of the fluid is then sent to a hospital laboratory to be checked for the presence of bacteria.

The doctor might also inject hydrocortisone, a steroid drug that has an anti-inflammatory effect, into the bursa. Once drained, the bursa is bandaged firmly. This treatment may have to be repeated a number of times before the effect becomes permanent.

Surgical removal

Surgical removal of the bursa involves cutting away as much of the fluid-forming sac as possible. The surgeon then clears out the accumulated clumps of clotted protein. This treatment is usually successful, although in a small minority of cases the bursa will form again in a few weeks.

Treatment of the impingement syndrome first involves strict rest from the activity that has caused the condition. It may be necessary for the sufferer to avoid all overhead movement of the arm for a period. The doctor will also prescribe drugs to control inflammation and fluid production and may have to inject steroids directly into the subachromial bursa. Once the pain has been relieved, an active physical therapy program is needed to restore full movement and to strengthen the muscles that control the rotator cuff.

There are various surgical procedures that can be used to reduce the pressure in the area under the shoulder blade (the subachromial space). This may involve removing part of the shoulder blade and part of the whole bursa.

Outlook

With treatment, acute bursitis usually clears up completely within a week or 10 days. If the cause is bacterial inflammation, the likelihood of recurrence is very rare.

Chronic bursitis usually recurs only if the rubbing or friction is repeated, so preventive measures are important. Thick clothing or padding of areas exposed to pressure is essential. Adequate seat cushioning helps prevent buttock bursas. To prevent prepatellar bursitis, knee pads are needed for jobs such as gardening or laying floors. Anyone who develops achillobursitis, inflammation in the Achilles tendon of the ankle, should avoid strenuous exercise.

The outlook in cases of the impingement syndrome depends on when treatment is given. If the condition has been neglected in the early stages, it may be necessary for the athlete to avoid all overhead movement permanently, but pain may persist despite this.

See also: Bacteria; Bunions; Inflammation; Joints; Painkillers; Physical therapy; Swellings; Tuberculosis

Calcium

Questions and Answers

I have heard that too much calcium is harmful. Would it be dangerous if I ate too much in my food?

No. The body regulates how much calcium it requires and absorbs the correct amount from your blood, if you eat an adequate diet. Excess calcium is passed out in the urine. However, taking too many vitamin D pills can upset the balance. If the absorption system goes wrong, kidney stones can result. A low-calcium diet helps to avoid this.

I am pregnant. Do I need calcium tablets to help my baby develop healthy bones and strong teeth?

No, not unless your diet is lacking in protein-rich food and fruit and vegetables. The intestine compensates for you and your baby's requirements and will absorb more calcium from your food as necessary. However, it does no harm to drink extra milk.

My grandmother, who is in her sixties, recently broke her arm in a minor accident. She believes that her bones have weakened since menopause. Is this possible?

Yes. The estrogen present in women before menopause helps build up calcium in the bones. After menopause, osteoporosis (thinning of the bones) may develop. Make sure that your grandmother has an adequate diet. Exercise, extra calcium, and biphosphonate drugs will also improve her condition.

How much milk should my three-year-old drink?

Three glasses of milk contain about 0.018 oz. (0.5 g) of calcium—an adequate daily intake for a one- to nine-year-old. There is calcium in other foods, so a balanced diet should provide enough calcium.

Calcium is essential to the human body—and it is present in amounts that are finely balanced so that we have neither too much nor too little. This balance can sometimes be upset, but treatment will correct the imbalance.

Bones and teeth contain a large proportion of calcium. Calcium crystals form solid building blocks that are held together by a fibrous network. The result is a strong, resilient material for supporting the body—bones. However, calcium is not permanently located in the bones, for it is constantly being mobilized to help maintain the correct levels in the body tissues elsewhere.

Small amounts of calcium regulate the impulses from the nerves in the brain and influence muscle contraction. Blood clotting also relies on a set amount of calcium in the blood.

Calcium balance

We absorb calcium from our food, and it passes, via the intestine, into the bloodstream. Some is lost in the urine. But some is stored in the bones or reabsorbed into the bloodstream.

A balanced level of calcium in the blood is maintained by an elaborate control system. This is located in the parathyroid glands in the neck. Their product, parathyroid hormone (PTH), acts on the bones and kidneys to release more calcium and also to decrease loss in the urine.

When calcium levels are low, more PTH is passed into the bloodstream, whereas high calcium levels will result in less PTH being sent out. In this way, a constant balance is maintained. Vitamin D is also essential for maintaining the balance of calcium. Without it, calcium cannot be absorbed from food. It also acts with PTH to release calcium from the bones.

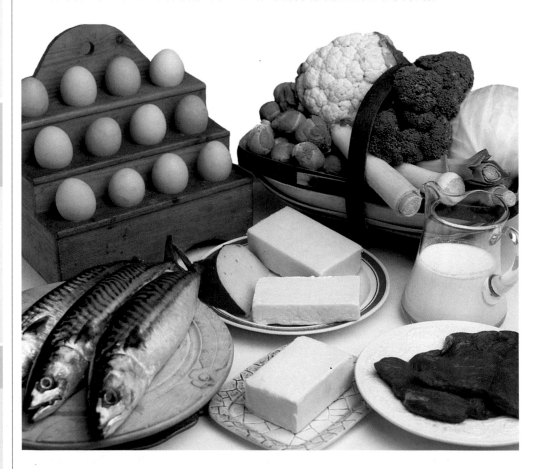

▲ *People need calcium to ensure, among other things, healthy bones and teeth. Calcium-rich foods include milk, cheese, eggs, meat, and vegetables.*

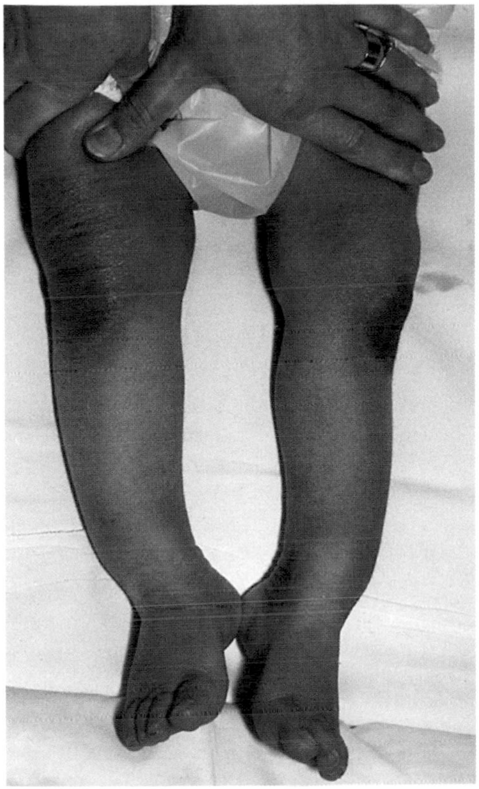

HOW THE BODY MAINTAINS A NORMAL CALCIUM BALANCE

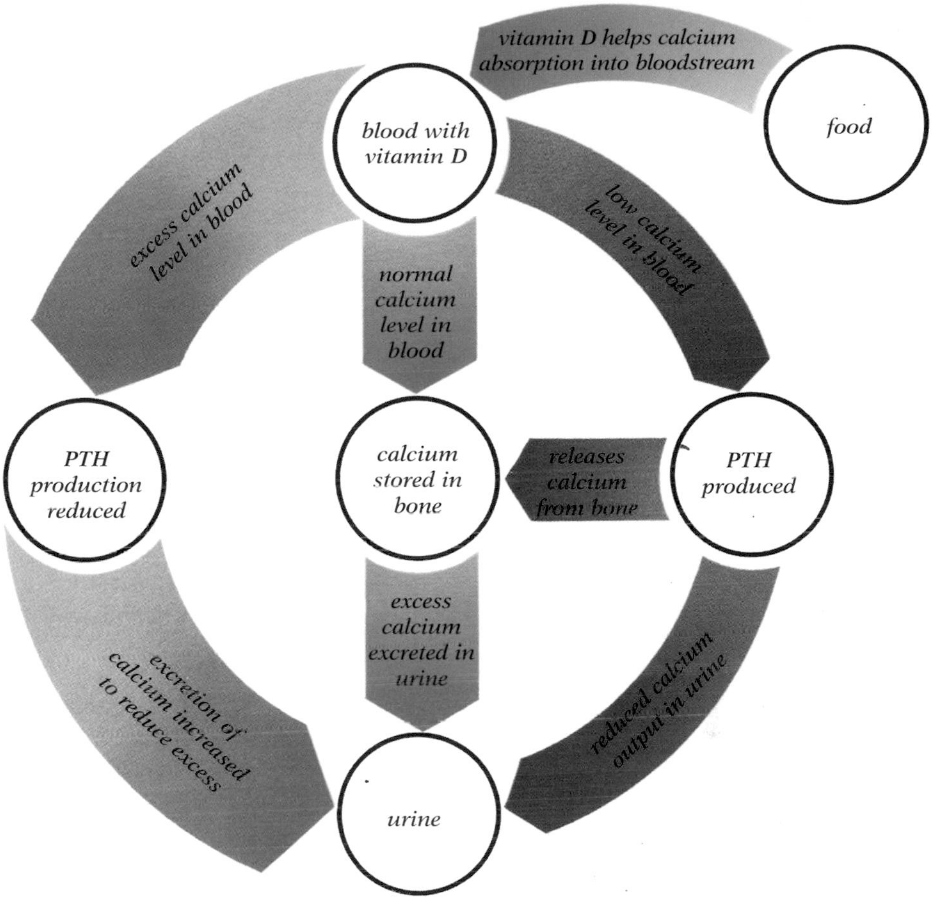

▲ This child has rickets, a bone condition caused by a deficiency of calcium and vitamin D—the leg bones are soft, so the legs bow outward.

vitamin D helps calcium absorption into bloodstream

food

blood with vitamin D

excess calcium level in blood

low calcium level in blood

normal calcium level in blood

PTH production reduced

calcium stored in bone

releases calcium from bone

PTH produced

excess calcium excreted in urine

excretion of calcium increased to reduce excess

reduced calcium output in urine

urine

Excessive calcium

If there is too much calcium in the body, vomiting and stomach pains may develop. Excess calcium may also be deposited in the kidneys and form renal stones (see Kidneys and Kidney Diseases). These are usually excreted naturally, but painfully. Too much calcium could be the result of a parathyroid tumor secreting uncontrolled amounts of PTH, or it could be that a person has taken too many vitamin D pills.

In an emergency, calcium levels can be reduced by phosphate injections or pills. A parathyroid tumor needs surgery. If the cause is vitamin pills, the patient must stop taking them.

A lack of calcium

If there is too little calcium, a condition known as tetany occurs—this describes spasms of the muscles, especially in the hands, feet, and larynx. One cause is hysterical overbreathing, triggered by fear or emotion, which temporarily reduces available blood calcium. As the hysteria passes, the body returns to normal.

If the parathyroid glands have to be removed, because of a tumor, for example, PTH levels can drop and cause tetany. This can be treated by giving intravenous calcium and oral vitamin D.

Low calcium can also produce abnormal blood clotting and unbalanced heart rhythms. However, muscle spasms occur first, so treatment can prevent other problems from developing.

If left untreated for months, loss of calcium from bones causes rickets in children, which results in bone deformities (see Rickets). In elderly people it causes osteoporosis (thinning bones; see

▲ Vitamin D is necessary for calcium to be absorbed from food. The level of calcium in the blood, which is controlled by PTH (parathyroid hormone), will be low if there is a lack of vitamin D. A lack of calcium in the blood causes PTH to be produced, and this encourages reduction of calcium stored in bones. Excess calcium in the blood reduces PTH production so that more calcium is excreted.

Osteoporosis). In both conditions, bones become weakened. Rickets still occurs today and can be helped by extra vitamin D. Many elderly women suffer from osteoporosis, largely because the loss of the anabolic steroid estrogen after menopause results in a progressive weakening of bones. The hormone calcitonin, given in pill form, is helpful to patients with osteoporosis (see Hormones).

Mother and baby

If a woman is pregnant or breast-feeding, her body loses calcium and vitamin D to the baby. Her intestine responds by absorbing more calcium and vitamin D from the food she eats. If she eats a balanced diet, there is no need for her to take calcium supplements (see Breast-feeding). If a mother is bottle-feeding her baby, the formula milk should be made as instructed, so that there is no calcium problem.

See also: Bones; Diet; Menopause; Muscles; Nervous system; Parathyroid glands; Pregnancy; Steroids; Teeth and teething; Vitamin D

Cancer

My brother has had a lot of X rays recently. Can these cause cancer?

The risk of developing cancer from X rays is so small as to be virtually insignificant. Doctors are aware of what risk there is and will advise you to have an X ray only if it is absolutely necessary.

Can cancer cells become resistant to the effects of chemotherapy (cytotoxic) drugs?

Unfortunately, yes. The reasons for this are uncertain, but after a while a cancer cell will find ways of reproducing itself despite the presence of the cytotoxic drug. Treatment must then be changed.

I have heard that interferons might cure many forms of cancer. Is this true?

Interferons are proteins produced by the body in response to viral infections. They have yielded only mixed results when used to treat cancers. While interferons are fairly promising against malignant melanoma and kidney cell cancer, and some lymphomas and leukemias, they show no potential for bowel, breast, or lung cancers. Their use to treat cancer can also induce serious side effects.

My aunt, who lives with us, has cancer. Is it infectious?

No. There is no risk of catching cancer from a relative or a friend with the disease.

Can wounds become cancerous?

Ulcers present for years may, very rarely, become cancerous. A cut or graze never does. However, a lump in the skin that ulcerates should be seen by a doctor, as, although ulcers rarely become cancerous, cancers often ulcerate.

Of all the medical conditions known, the one that creates the most fear in people today is cancer. In fact, in many cases early diagnosis and continually improving forms of treatment can mean a complete cure.

Cancer is the result of disordered and disorganized cell growth. This can be fully understood only by looking at what happens in normal cells. The human body is made up of many different tissues—for example, skin, lung, and liver—in turn made up of millions of cells. These are all arranged in an orderly manner, each individual tissue having its own cellular structure. In addition, the appearance and shape of the cells of one organ differ from those of another. For example, a liver cell and skin cell look completely different (see Cells and Chromosomes).

In all tissues, cells are constantly being lost through general wear and tear. They are replaced by a process of cell division, occurring so that exactly the right number of cells are produced to replace those that are lost. A normal cell will divide in half to create two new cells, each identical to the original. If the body is injured, the rate of cell production speeds up automatically until the injury is healed, when it slows down again.

The cells of a cancer, however, divide and grow at their own speed, in an uncontrolled manner. They continue to do so indefinitely unless treatment is given. In time, the cancer cells increase in numbers until enough are present for the cancer to become visible as a growth.

In addition to growing too rapidly, cancer cells are unable to organize themselves properly, so the mass of tissue that forms is not like normal tissue. Cancer gets its nourishment parasitically from its host and serves no useful purpose in the body.

Cancers are classified according to the cell from which they originated. Those that arise from cells in the surface membranes of the body (the epithelial tissues), like the skin and the lining of the lungs and gastrointestinal tract, are called carcinomas. Those arising from structures deep inside the body, such as bone cartilage and muscle, are known as sarcomas. Carcinomas are much more common than sarcomas. This may be because the cells of the surface membranes need to divide more often in order to keep these membranes intact.

Benign and malignant tumors

Not all tumors are cancerous. Although tumor cells grow at their own speed, tumors can be benign or malignant (see Tumors). Benign tumors push aside normal tissues but do not grow into them. Malignant tumors (cancers), grow into surrounding tissue, a process called invasion. It is this clawlike process of abnormal cells permeating normal tissues that gives the name

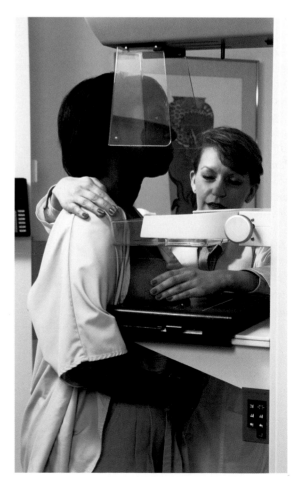

▶ *This patient is undergoing a mammogram, which is an X ray of the breast to screen for cancer and to investigate lumps in the breast.*

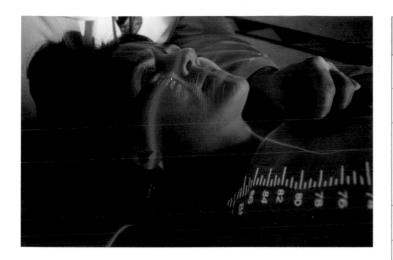

▲ *This woman is receiving laser radiation treatment, which damages the genetic material of cancer cells.*

Steps you can take regarding cancer
Stop smoking and drink alcohol in moderation.
Examine your breasts or testicles once a month for lumps.
If you are a woman, have a cervical (Pap) smear done at least once a year.
Eat a balanced diet.
Avoid sunburn, particularly if you have a fair complexion.
See your doctor if you develop symptoms such as persistent pain, bleeding, or a lump.

cancer—from a zodiacal constellation, the crab. Its invasive properties enable unchecked cancer to spread through the body. The word malignant means "bad," while benign means "harmless." A benign tumor can look almost like normal tissue under the microscope, and it behaves accordingly, respecting its neighbors. It also grows more slowly than a malignant tumor. Although usually harmless, a benign tumor can be serious if it arises in an important part of the body, such as the brain cavity. An important difference between benign and malignant tumors is that the latter can seed themselves to start up in remote parts of the body (a process called metastasis); benign tumors never do this. Benign tumors should be removed, and surgery is nearly always curative.

Origin of cancer cells

Cancer cells develop from the body's own normal cells, and a single cancer cell is enough to start the growth of a tumor. However, the change to a cancer cell is a gradual one, taking place in stages over several years. With each stage the cell becomes slightly more abnormal in appearance and slightly less responsive to the body's control mechanisms. This process is usually unseen until a cancer develops, but in a few cases precancer can be recognized and treated. The best precancer known is seen in the uterine cervix, the neck of the womb, and this can be detected by a Pap smear (see Cervix and Cervical Smears).

How cancer spreads

The abnormal growth of a cancer is localized, at least at first, forming a mass around the original cells. However, the cancer usually invades normal tissues very early. If these tissues are important, life and health may be threatened.

The feature of cancer that accounts for most of its devastating effects is its ability to spread, or metastasize, to other parts of the body. Metastasis does not usually occur until the original collection of cells has grown to a fair size. Science does not yet fully understand the biological processes of metastasis, but evidence exists that single cancer cells, or small clumps, break off from the main cancer and are carried to other areas of the body by the blood or lymphatic system (see Lymphatic System). Cancer cells carried by the blood are thought first to enter capillaries or very small veins or arteries. They travel until they come to a place where the blood vessels divide to form channels so small that the cancer cells cannot easily get through. At that point they may lodge and begin to grow, producing a new cancer mass. The first place this is likely to occur is the liver, for most cancers of the gastrointestinal tract; or the lungs, for most cancers starting elsewhere in the body. This is because these organs are the first places where blood from other organs is filtered through a network of minute blood vessels. Thus, the lungs and liver are the most common sites of metastasis from blood-borne cancer cells. However, the cells can also pass through the liver and lungs to lodge in other regions of the body—often in the bones or structures of the head and trunk.

Normal lymph drainage begins in the peripheral lymphatic vessels, proceeding through a sequence of small structures called lymph nodes, and finally reaching one of the large central veins. These nodes, which serve as filters, contain many tiny channels through which the lymph and any cancer cells or other foreign matter must pass. Cancer cells that manage to pass through the lymph nodes and enter the bloodstream probably metastasize in the same way as cells that enter the blood directly.

Causes

The immune system is able to detect cells that have developed cancerous changes. Most of these cells are quickly attacked and destroyed by immune system cells. If it were not for this form of surveillance, cancer would be almost universal. There are, however, limits to the efficiency of the system. Cancer is most common in late middle age and old age. The increasing frequency of cancer in the Western world may, in part, be because people are living longer, but some cancers are associated with the Western way of life itself. Cancers due to smoking, for example, are still less common in the developing world. Nonetheless, the speed with which people are taking up smoking in these regions will ensure a high prevalence of cancers within a decade or two. The most common forms are lung, bowel, stomach, pancreas, and breast cancer. Despite developments in modern medicine, these cancers still account for many deaths in the United States each year. The most common cancers in children and young adults are leukemias, sarcomas, and kidney cancer. These cancers are rare, and their treatment has improved in recent years.

Questions and Answers

My uncle has had radiotherapy once and has now been told he has to have a second course of treatment. Is this safe?

Not if it is given to the same part of the body, unless it is a very small dose. However, the doctor will know how much radiotherapy a part of your uncle's body will tolerate. He or she will advise a second treatment only if it is safe. It is possible to give a full course of treatment to a different body part.

Can cancer ever be hereditary?

Not usually. There are a few cancers that run in families, but they are rare. Only if cancer is particularly common in your family is there any increased risk. If this is so, take better care of yourself, and report any persistent symptoms to your doctor.

I have been smoking up to 60 cigarettes a day and am worried about cancer. How many should I cut down to to be safe?

You are right to be worried. You do not say how many years you have been smoking, but it could be that you have damaged your lungs irreversibly—though this damage may not be cancerous. As far as cutting down is concerned, the advice can be summed up in two words—quit altogether!

I have read that cancer is sometimes stress-related. Also I have an aunt who literally willed herself to live against all odds. With cancer, can it ever be a case of mind over matter?

This is an interesting question. There are cases where the fear of getting cancer, often when one person in a family already has the disease, seems to bring it on in other members of the family. So perhaps fear does act as a trigger. In the same way, sheer determination has been known to get individuals out of the worst situations, as your aunt's case seems to indicate. The answer is that no one really knows for sure.

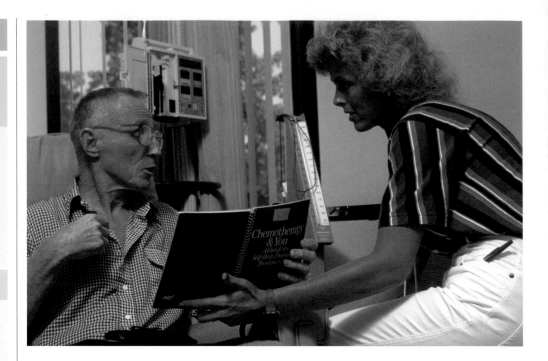

▲ *Chemotherapy, the use of cytotoxic drugs, may be a cancer treatment on its own or it may be combined with surgery, radiotherapy, or both.*

The cause of cancer is unknown, but two fundamental abnormalities are recognized. First, cancers are not subject to the normal influences that control cell growth. Second, the body will tolerate the presence of the cancer without rejecting it as a foreign invader. Environmental factors, such as chemical pollution and exposure to radiation, are thought to lead to cancer, but there are several other factors at work. Some cancers are known to be caused by viruses (oncoviruses) that can inject cancer-causing genes (oncogenes) into the DNA of normal cells.

Certain chemicals can also cause cells to become cancerous. These chemicals are irritants that may alter a cell's genetic structure and turn it into a cancer cell. Experiments have identified chemicals that cause cancer in animals (carcinogens). The best-known carcinogens are some of the 3,000 or so different chemicals present in tobacco smoke (see Smoking). However, despite research, it has not yet been possible to identify the carcinogens responsible for many common cancers. As no single theory explains all the facts about cancer, it seems probable that cancer has many causes, some of which are still unknown (see Viruses).

Pap smear

Cancer may be discovered because it causes symptoms, or it may be found by screening. The earlier a cancer is detected, the higher the chance of a cure. Much research has been done on developing screening examinations to detect cancer early. The greatest success has been the Pap test to detect carcinoma in the cervix. The test is effective, quick, simple, and inexpensive. A few cells are scraped off the cervix, put on a microscope slide, dyed, and examined. Any cancerous cells can sometimes be destroyed without having to remove the uterus. If this is not possible, surgical removal of the uterus at this stage results in complete cure of the carcinoma.

Cancer screening

Screening examinations of women without symptoms are also effective for the early detection of breast cancer, especially for women over the age of 50. A yearly combination of physical examination, study of medical history, and mammography—a special X-ray test—can reduce mortality from breast cancer in this age group by at least one-third.

Regular screening is also recommended as early as age 35 for women who have a mother or sister with this kind of cancer and for those who have already had breast cancer. In addition, two breast cancer genes, BRCA I and BRCA II, have now been identified. These occur in a small category of women whose tendency to breast cancer is significantly higher than normal. These women will also require close follow-up (see Mammography).

Two methods exist for detecting cancer of the colon and rectum before symptoms occur—careful medical examination and tests for small amounts of blood in the feces.

Doctors and others have also proposed screening for some other kinds of cancer, especially for persons known to be at high risk. However, it is currently felt that extensive screening of the general population is not advisable, because of the high costs of such tests, the low yield of unsuspected cancers, and the lack of evidence that survival rates would improve.

Diagnosis

It is no longer true that cancer is always fatal. There has been a vast improvement in the treatment of cancer in recent years, and many thousands of people are cured of the disease each year. However, a small cancer is easier to cure than a large one, so early diagnosis is vital and is helped by the prompt reporting of significant symptoms to a doctor. If the doctor suspects the possibility of cancer, he or she will refer the patient to a specialist.

The specialist will first confirm the diagnosis. This may initially involve X rays (such as a mammography) and scanning tests to show if there is a lump present. A part of the tissue will then be examined under the microscope. This can be done either by biopsy or by cytological examination. A biopsy involves a surgeon removing a small piece of the tumor, which is then sent to a pathologist for examination (see Biopsy). This will determine whether the suspected tissue is cancerous or not. In a cytological examination, body fluids, such as mucus from the uterine cervix, are studied specifically for cancer cells (see Pap Smear).

The specialist will also carry out a thorough examination of the patient, taking particular care to check the lymph nodes adjacent to the tumor. He or she will also run blood tests to check liver and bone function and will arrange a chest X ray to look for evidence of spread into these sites. If the doctor suspects that cancer has spread to a particular part of the body, this area may also be scanned.

Various scanning techniques are used. In isotope scanning, a tiny amount of radioactive substance is injected into the body, and blood then carries it to the suspected organ or area of tissue. If the tissue contains a cancer, this will take up a different amount of isotope compared with the rest of the healthy tissue. The patient is then scanned with a special instrument that detects the radiation, and the cancer can be seen. Bones and the liver are the most common areas to be scanned in this way (see Diagnostic Imaging; Scans).

The doctor now has a detailed knowledge of the type of cancer involved and the stage of its development. Using this information, he or she can decide on the form of treatment that is most likely to be effective. The aim of all cancer treatment is to kill or remove every cancer cell. This is often possible.

Surgery

Cancer surgery aims at removing all of the cancer from the patient. It usually involves removing the visible growth with a wide margin of surrounding normal tissue to make sure every cell is taken. In addition, the surgeon will remove the draining lymph nodes and examine any adjacent structures. After removing the tumor, the surgeon will, where possible, reconstruct the patient's anatomy.

Nonetheless, patterns of surgery in breast cancer have changed in recent years to become more conservative. Research has shown that the long-term survival rate of women with small breast cancers

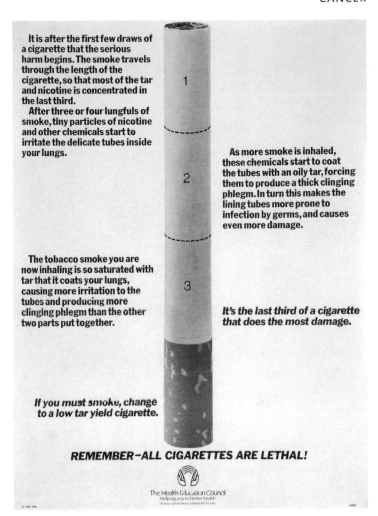

It is after the first few draws of a cigarette that the serious harm begins. The smoke travels through the length of the cigarette, so that most of the tar and nicotine is concentrated in the last third.

After three or four lungfuls of smoke, tiny particles of nicotine and other chemicals start to irritate the delicate tubes inside your lungs.

As more smoke is inhaled, these chemicals start to coat the tubes with an oily tar, forcing them to produce a thick clinging phlegm. In turn this makes the lining tubes more prone to infection by germs, and causes even more damage.

The tobacco smoke you are now inhaling is so saturated with tar that it coats your lungs, causing more irritation to the tubes and producing more clinging phlegm than the other two parts put together.

It's the last third of a cigarette that does the most damage.

If you must smoke, change to a low tar yield cigarette.

REMEMBER—ALL CIGARETTES ARE LETHAL!

The Health Education Council
Helping you to better health

▲ *This poster emphasizes the dangers of smoking and reminds people that smoking is lethal.*

who undergo limited operations such as "lumpectomy" (in which only the discernible lump is removed), or breast-conserving surgery, is the same as in those who undergo complete breast removal.

There are some circumstances in which surgery is carried out without investigating the patient first. Obviously, when the patient is presented as an emergency, surgery is performed both to diagnose and to treat the patient.

There are also some situations when a biopsy and a cancer operation are carried out under the same anesthetic. For example, it used to be common practice to biopsy a breast lump, examine the tissue, and to then perform more extensive surgery if the lump was found to be malignant (see Pathology).

However, most breast biopsies are now done using a fine needle technique under local anesthetic. This leaves no scar and does not require hospital admission. It also permits the patient to participate in decisions about her treatment before surgery.

Radiotherapy

The aim of radiotherapy is to destroy the cancer with irradiation. Radiation damages the genetic material of cancer cells, so that they are unable to divide. Because they divide more rapidly than normal cells, cancer cells are more sensitive than normal cells to the damaging effects of radiation. Normal cells are also liable to be

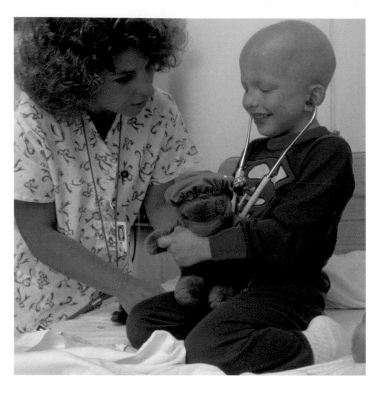

▲ *This nine-year-old girl is suffering from acute lymphoblastic leukemia (a cancer of the blood). Treatment includes a two-year course of chemotherapy, which has caused her hair to fall out.*

hair usually regrows within six months. Damage to other parts of the body is now rare, since the dosage that sensitive organs, such as the kidneys and lungs, will tolerate is known, and this dose is not exceeded (see Radiation Sickness; Radiotherapy).

Radiotherapy is used for localized tumors in addition to surgery. Some cancers—for example, some of the head and neck—can be cured by radiotherapy without surgery. In other cases, radiotherapy can be given either before or after an operation to increase the chances of success—as with breast cancer, for example.

Radioactive implants

In some circumstances it is actually possible to implant radioactive substances in the cancer. These give a very large dose to the cancer itself with only a small dose to the surrounding normal tissue. This form of treatment is ideal, as the damage to normal tissues is minimal. Unfortunately, it is possible only in accessible tumors, such as small cancers of the tongue and mouth and some that are gynecological in nature. Radiotherapy is also very good at relieving the symptoms of incurable cancer, particularly pain.

Chemotherapy

If a cancer is too widespread or metastases are present, it may not be possible to use radiotherapy effectively. Doctors can prescribe drug

damaged by radiation, but it is the difference in the rate of reproduction between cancer cells and normal cells that makes radiotherapy both possible and valuable.

Radiotherapy is given in special rooms with thick floors, walls, ceilings, and windows to prevent radiation leaks. The patient lies on a special couch beneath the machine, and the machine is aimed at the tumor. Before treatment, the radiotherapist takes careful measurements of the position of the tumor to work out the best angle or combination of angles at which to set the machine. The staff leave the room before the machine is switched on. It is essential that the patient is in exactly the same position for every treatment. The treatment lasts only a few minutes and is painless—it is usually given daily for five to six weeks on an outpatient basis.

Side effects of radiotherapy can be kept to a minimum by careful medical supervision. Soreness of the skin is less of a problem today and may be avoided by infrequent washing of the treatment area. Soothing creams are also given to the patient. Sickness and diarrhea are problems only when the abdomen is treated, and they can usually be controlled with drugs. Loss of hair may occur if the head is treated, but

Symptoms of common cancers

TYPE	SYMPTOMS
Breast cancer	Breast lump, bleeding from the nipple, inverted nipple, change in the shape of the breast.
Cancer of the larynx	Persistent hoarseness, spitting up blood.
Cancer of the esophagus (gullet)	Difficulty in swallowing, vomiting, loss of weight.
Cancer of the stomach	Difficulty in swallowing, vomiting, bringing up blood, loss of weight, indigestion.
Cancer of the bowel	Blood in the feces or from the rectum, a change of bowel habit—either constipation or diarrhea, or abdominal pain.
Cancer of the bladder	Blood in the urine.
Cancer of the prostate	Increased difficulty in passing urine; recurring urinary infections and back pain.
Cancer of the uterus or cervix	If menstruating, bleeding in between periods; if postmenopausal, vaginal bleeding. Offensive-smelling vaginal discharge, lower abdominal pain.
Cancer of the mouth and throat	Sore ulcer that refuses to heal; pain in ear or ears; difficulty in chewing or swallowing; dentures do not fit.
Leukemia	Tiredness, pallor, repeated infections, sore throat, bleeding from gums and nose, bruising.
Lung cancer	Persistent cough, spitting up blood, shortness of breath, chest pain, hoarseness.
Skin cancer	Sore skin that will not heal and continually bleeds.

Differences between benign and malignant tumors

TYPE OF GROWTH	BENIGN Pushes normal tissue aside.	MALIGNANT Invades normal tissue.
Spread	Slight.	May form secondary growths.
Structure	Similar to normal growths.	May be disorganized.
Rate	Slow.	May be slow to rapid.
Outcome	Usually harmless.	May be fatal if untreated.
Treatment	Surgery is curative.	Surgery may not be curative.

Hormones are chemical messengers that circulate in the blood to control the growth and metabolism of tissue (see Hormones). If a cancer cell arises in a hormone-sensitive organ, such as the uterus (womb), it may continue to recognize and respond to hormonal messages. If the patient is then given an inhibitory hormone—one that tells the cells to stop dividing—the cancer will stop growing. This treatment is particularly useful in breast, uterine, and prostate cancers. Its great advantage is its freedom from unpleasant side effects.

treatment in this situation. The drugs combine with and damage the genetic material of cells so that they cannot divide properly. Historically, the earliest chemotherapeutic agents were developed from mustard gas. Doctors noticed that soldiers recovering from this poisoning had low blood counts. They quickly realized that the gas was interfering with the division of cells in the bone marrow, where blood is made. Nitrogen mustard (the active drug in mustard gas) was tried in cancer patients in an attempt to poison the cancer cells, and it proved successful. Many new, safer drugs have since been discovered, and effective combinations of drugs have been developed. Unfortunately, these drugs poison all dividing cells. The best way to minimize the damage to normal cells is to give fewer, larger doses of cytotoxic (cell poisoning) drugs over a short period of time. There is then a gap of a few weeks (usually three) before the next course of treatment. This allows normal cells to recover.

Side effects of cancer treatment
The possible side effects of cytotoxic drugs—or chemotherapy, as these are now called—include hair loss, nausea, and lowering of the blood count. Hair loss occurs with a few of the cytotoxic drugs, but the hair regrows when treatment stops. Nausea sometimes follows the injection of some cytotoxic drugs but usually lasts only a few hours. Drugs that combat nausea can be prescribed.

Alternatively, when nausea is severe, the patient may be admitted to a hospital and the treatment given under sedation. However, this is rarely necessary. The safe dosage for the various cytotoxic drugs is now known to doctors, so serious depression of the patient's blood count is now a much rarer occurrence than it used to be. However, the blood must be regularly tested both before and during drug treatment.

Chemotherapy is not used solely for solid-tissue tumors. It is also used to treat blood cancers, such as leukemia, as it has proved effective on bone marrow (see Leukemia).

Other cancers, such as Hodgkin's disease, may respond better to a treatment like chemotherapy rather than to extensive radiotherapy (see Hodgkin's Disease). In some cases where the patient has tended to relapse after surgery or radiotherapy, chemotherapy is given even when there is no sign of cancer.

This treatment is called adjuvant chemotherapy and is being tried for breast cancer and childhood cancer. Although encouraging results have been obtained, it is still too early to advocate this kind of treatment for all cancer patients.

Blocking hormone action
Prostate cancers are usually encouraged by testosterone and can be effectively treated either by removal of the testosterone source (the testicles) or by the use of a drug such as bicalutamine (Casodex), which blocks the action of testosterone. Many breast cancers are encouraged by estrogen and can be helped, or possibly prevented, by the drug tamoxifen, which blocks the action of estrogens.

Combined treatment
Where more than one cancer therapy has been found to be effective, treatments may be combined. In some childhood tumors, for example, surgery is followed by local radiotherapy and then one year of chemotherapy. In head and neck cancer, chemotherapy is followed by local radiotherapy, and then any of the tumor that still remains is removed surgically. Much research is now being carried out to determine the best possible way of combining treatments.

Whole-body irradiation and bone-marrow transplantation
In recent years it has become possible to transplant bone marrow from one person to another. This specialized procedure requires that large doses of radiation be given to the recipient beforehand—an approach called whole-body irradiation. At present this treatment is generally used only for rare forms of anemia and leukemia. In the future, however, it may be possible to treat other forms of cancer in this way.

Outlook
Many cancers are curable if they are treated early enough, so regular screening is important for early diagnosis and treatment. Any persistent or unexplained symptoms must be reported to a doctor. Once the treatment has been completed, the doctor will regularly examine the original cancer site with care, and he or she will also investigate any new symptoms that appear. If the patient is still well and free of cancer five years later, there is room for cautious optimism.

Recent advances made in medical research, and subsequently treatment, are getting better all the time—as are the chances of surviving cancer.

See also: Anemia; Bones; Immune system; Liver and liver diseases; Lung and lung diseases; Mastectomy; Photosensitivity; Screening; Surgery; X rays

Capillaries

Questions and Answers

I have recently developed some odd, purple patches on my skin. What can they be?

The spontaneous appearance of purple patches on the skin always calls for medical attention. The most likely cause is a condition known as purpura, where the capillaries leak blood into the skin. In older people this may be due to loss of collagen support for the fine vessels. However, the condition may also be caused by a drop in the number of blood platelets, which assist in the clot formation necessary to plug small openings in blood vessels. Purpura may be a minor problem but can indicate a serious bleeding disorder.

I have always bruised easily. Do I have weak capillaries?

Yes. The walls of your capillaries could be more fragile than usual, but this is nothing to worry about. You should see a doctor only if you get a crop of tiny bruises without any injury, as these can be a sign that something is wrong with your blood.

Why does drinking alcohol make my face turn pink?

Alcohol dilates the capillaries of the skin. Rapid temperature changes can have the same effect. If this happens often, the capillaries can become permanently stretched, resulting in a pinkness of the skin that does not die down. The best way to prevent this is to avoid excessive alcohol and temperature changes.

Do capillaries occur in all parts of the body?

Yes. Capillaries are essential as the interface between the blood and the tissues and occur everywhere. No part of the body, even the bones, is free from capillaries.

The capillaries are the smallest blood vessels and form a complex network throughout the body. In addition to carrying oxygen and other vital substances to and from cells, they also help regulate body temperature.

The capillaries form an extensive network of vessels between the arterial system, which takes the blood from the heart, and the venous system, which returns the blood to the heart (see Circulatory System). Each capillary measures only about 0.0003 inch (0.008 mm), or only just wider than one single blood cell. The capillaries' job—one of the most essential in the human body—is to deliver oxygen and other vital substances to the cells and to collect the cells' waste products, which they do through their thin walls.

Structure

Capillaries are simple structures and their walls consist of little more than a single layer of very thin, flattened cells called endothelial cells, which are connected together edge to edge. Each capillary consists of a thin layer of tissue rolled up into a tube and surrounded by an equally thin membrane. All the capillary walls are thin enough to allow certain substances to pass in and out of the blood.

Electron microscopy has shown that in different locations throughout the body, capillary structure varies widely. Those in the kidneys, the lining of the intestines, the endocrine glands, and the pancreas, for instance, are perforated by tiny pores of widely differing size.

Those in the brain differ considerably from those in the rest of the body, especially in thickness. Their thicker walls provide what is known as the blood-brain barrier. This is an effective obstruction to the passage of certain drugs and other substances from the blood to the brain

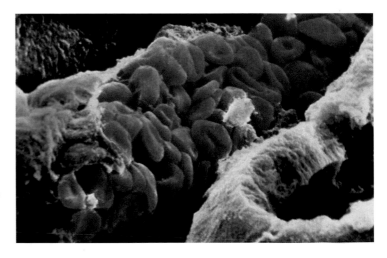

▶ ▼ *A capillary (right). Transfer of substances from blood to surrounding tissues happens as shown below: water, food molecules, and hormones go through pores; oxygen and carbon dioxide are exchanged via walls; and protein molecules are engulfed by capillary walls, then released outside.*

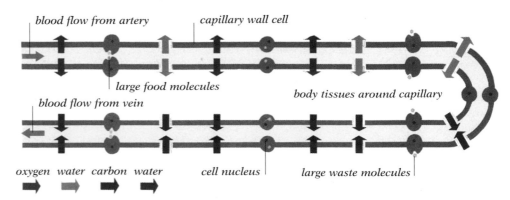

blood flow from artery   capillary wall cell

large food molecules

blood flow from vein   body tissues around capillary

oxygen water carbon water   cell nucleus   large waste molecules

cells and the cerebrospinal fluid (the fluid that surrounds the brain). This barrier offers protection for the brain against many potentially damaging substances commonly found in the blood, but it does have the disadvantage that it can interfere with treatment from antibiotics and other drugs. Doses of antibiotics for the brain may have to be increased to many times those that are needed for infections elsewhere in the body (see Blood-Brain Barrier).

Connecting link

As the heart pumps blood through the body, the blood goes first through the arteries. The arteries divide into branches called arterioles. The branches become smaller and smaller, and the smallest are the capillaries. In the capillaries the blood cells jostle along in single file, giving up oxygen, nutrients, and other substances, and taking in carbon dioxide and other waste products from the cells. When this process is finished, the blood needs to return to the heart. As this return journey starts, the capillaries join up to form small veins that gradually grow larger as many branches join them.

When the body is at rest, blood flows through preferential, or preferred, channels. These are capillaries that have become larger than average. However, when extra oxygen is needed by a particular part of the body—for example, by the muscles or the heart during exercise—blood flows through nearly all the capillaries in that area.

Capillary gaps

All capillaries have small gaps between the edges of the cells that form their walls. These gaps are very important. The pressure of the blood in the capillaries is low, but it is highest at the arterial end of any capillary (the part through which blood enters the capillary) and lowest at the venous end (the part through which blood leaves the capillary). As a result, some of the watery part of the blood, but not the red cells or large protein molecules, passes out through the gaps and pores in the capillary walls at the arterial end. Most of this fluid passes back in through the walls at the venous end of the capillary.

Outside the capillaries, this fluid is called tissue fluid. It bathes the cells of the body, allowing diffusion of important dissolved substances from the blood to the cells, and from the cells to the blood. This is how oxygen, nutrients, vitamins, minerals, hormones, and so on are able to get to the cells from the blood, and how waste products of cell metabolism are carried away from the cells to be disposed of via the bloodstream (see Blood).

There is another important reason for the gaps in the capillary walls. Although they are too small to allow red blood cells to pass, cells capable of changing their shape can do so. Such cells are said to be ameboid, and they pass through the capillary wall gaps in a remarkable way. First the cell pushes a tiny finger through a gap. The substance of the cell then flows along this finger and expands outside the capillary. This process continues until the whole of the cell is outside. Called phagocytes, cells of this kind belong to the immune system. Their function is to combat infection, and millions of them pass through capillary walls at the site of any inflammation.

Sinusoids

There is one particular class of capillaries that differs from all other capillaries. These are known as the sinusoids. The sinusoids are of wider caliber and are more irregular than other capillaries, but the most striking difference is the number and size of the openings in their walls. The sinusoids in the liver have numerous relatively large

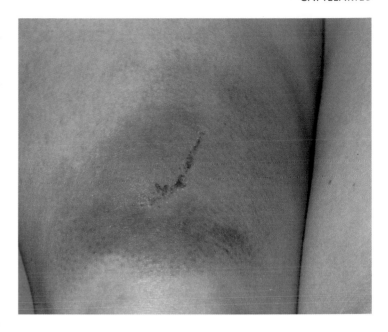

▲ *If the skin receives a heavy blow—in the case above a kick from a horse—the capillaries in the skin's surface break and release their blood. This released blood causes the skin to discolor and form a bruise.*

openings grouped so as to form sieve plates. Those in the spleen have long, slitlike openings in their walls that, unlike capillaries anywhere else in the body, allow whole blood to pass through into the surrounding space.

Regulating body temperature

In addition to the exchange of substances, the capillaries located in the skin play a special role—they help to regulate body temperature. When the body is hot, the capillaries in the skin get wider, making it possible for a larger volume of blood to reach the skin, where it can be cooled by the outside air. Capillaries widen and narrow passively as a result of changes in the pressure of the blood within them. This, in turn, is determined by the flow rate in the tiny arterioles supplying the capillaries. Arterioles have muscle fibers in their walls, which can tighten to narrow the vessels or relax to widen them. The muscles in the walls of the arterioles are under the control of the autonomic nervous system and the endocrine system.

Damage to capillaries

Since they are thin-walled, capillaries are easily damaged. Those most at risk are the capillaries in the skin. If the skin is scratched, cut, or injured, or if it receives a blow, the capillaries release blood. A bruise results as blood collects in the skin (see Bruises). Capillaries can also be damaged or destroyed by burning, but they have some ability to renew themselves. As a person grows older, or as the result of drinking excess alcohol over a long period of time, the capillaries collapse, leaving visible purple patches or a network of reddish lines on the skin of the face.

> *See also:* Antibiotics; Cells and chromosomes; Endocrine system; Exercise; Immune system; Inflammation; Nervous system; Veins; Vitamins

Cardiac massage

Cardiac massage is one method used to stimulate the heart into action when it has stopped beating. The technique can restore breathing and circulation and save a life if applied correctly.

Questions and Answers

How much time should elapse after cardiac arrest before cardiac massage is given?

Cardiac arrest is a medical emergency. Nothing should delay restoring the blood circulation. You should not, for instance, waste time trying to feel for a pulse. This is difficult to do and may be misleading, as you may be feeling your own pulse. Lack of blood flow to the brain for three or four minutes usually results in brain damage. Although you might be able to get the heart beating again, the patient might die from the brain damage. Even if the patient lives, there may be permanent mental impairment. If more than 10 minutes goes by before resuscitation is begun, the brain will be irreparably damaged.

What should be done if a person has a cardiac arrest while eating and the mouth is filled with food?

Since cardiac massage and mouth-to-mouth resuscitation are given together, it is important that there is no obstruction to the airways while the latter is being performed. To remove any food from the person's mouth and throat, tilt the head back and sideways, pull or push the jaw out, and move the tongue from the back of the throat. Close the nostrils with your fingers and blow strongly into the patient's mouth on every fifteenth chest compression. If the chest does not expand, food may still be left in the throat, or your technique is faulty. Chest compressions usually clear any obstructions.

If I saw someone collapse in the street, how would I know whether he or she was in cardiac arrest?

If the person is unconscious, check briefly to see if he or she is breathing. If the pupils are dilated and the skin is turning gray, start cardiac massage immediately.

Cardiac massage, or cardiac compression, is the first-aid technique used to stimulate blood flow from the heart by pressing on the patient's chest wall. External cardiac compression (ECC) is always given together with expired air resuscitation (the kiss of life): the two together are called cardiopulmonary resuscitation (CPR).

Cardiac compression is given in cases of cardiac arrest, when the normal rhythmic beating of the heart becomes disturbed and the heart's contractions stop. Cardiac arrest can be caused by various factors: drowning, asphyxiation, hemorrhaging, electrocution, drug overdose, cardiac infarction (blocking of blood circulation), coronary air embolism (an air bubble in a vein that reaches the heart), and pulmonary embolism (an obstruction of the pulmonary artery by a blood clot).

Signs of cardiac arrest

Although an electrocardiogram (ECG)—a test that shows the pattern of heartbeats on a graph—is needed to detect whether the heart has actually stopped, there are certain signs indicating that a patient is experiencing cardiac arrest and circulatory failure. About six to 12 seconds after the heart has stopped, the patient will lose consciousness. No pulse will be felt. Fifteen to 30 seconds after circulation has ceased, breathing will stop. The skin will turn gray, and the pupils will become dilated. If there is breathing, coughing, spontaneous movement, or movement in response to any stimulus, the person is not in cardiac arrest.

If the signs of cardiac arrest are present, however, resuscitation is urgently required to restart circulation and breathing. There is only a maximum of ten minutes in which to do this. Within three or four minutes after circulation ceases, the heart will become damaged because of lack of oxygen. Although the heart may be restarted, the brain will suffer irreversible damage.

Blood flow

The principle of cardiac massage is that rhythmic compression of the chest wall can replace the action of the heart muscle and generate blood flow in the carotid arteries. These arteries supply blood to the brain to resuscitate it. What happens to the heart and to the blood flow during external compression is that, as the resuscitator squeezes down, blood is driven from the heart and from all the large vessels within the chest. Backward flow of blood is prevented by valves at the point where the great veins of the head enter the chest (see Heart).

The chest therefore can be thought of as a large sponge full of blood that is emptied by one massive squeezing motion, which is sustained for about half a second. At this point the aortic valve, which stands between the aorta (supplying blood to the whole body) and the left ventricle (the main pump from which the blood to the body comes), slams shut and prevents all the pumped blood from flowing backward into the heart. During relaxation, the sponge reexpands and blood runs back to fill the spaces formed. With the next squeeze of the sponge, blood is further driven forward. The process is then repeated.

Performing cardiac compression

In case of cardiac arrest, heart massage should be started immediately. No special equipment is necessary, nor is the help of a doctor required.

The patient should be laid on his or her back on a hard surface. The person performing the cardiac massage should make no attempt to check whether a pulse is present. In the circumstances it may be extremely difficult to feel a pulse. In 40 percent of cases a faint pulse cannot be reliably felt, and in 10 percent a pulse is thought to be present when there is no heart action.

To find the correct place for the massage, a hand should be moved down the patient's chest to the lower third part of the sternum (breastbone) and the fingers placed at the point where the patient's ribs join, on a line midway between the nipples; there is often a small bone here called

FIRST AID FOR CARDIAC ARREST

HEART MASSAGE COMBINED WITH THE "KISS OF LIFE"

When someone is unconscious, the first thing to do is to evaluate the patient's condition. If the patient is not breathing or if his or her heart has stopped, or if there is severe bleeding, immediate action is required. First, contact the emergency services, then do what you can. Loosen the patient's clothing and check that the airways are clear by running your finger inside the patient's mouth. Look for movement of any kind, breathing, or coughing. Only trained first aiders should check for a pulse before beginning chest compressions.

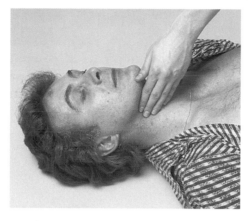

Lay the patient on his or her back on a hard surface. If you are skilled in first aid, feel for the carotid pulse in the neck to one side of the Adam's apple.

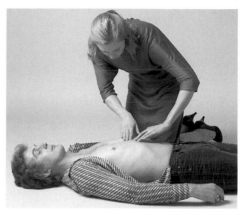

Establish the position of the heart by running your fingers down the chest to the lower third part of the breastbone. Place them at the point where the ribs join (you may feel a small bone).

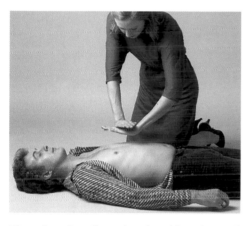

Place the palm of your hand at this point, and the palm of your other hand on top of it. Press vertically downward, rhythmically, 60 times a minute. Try to keep your elbows straight.

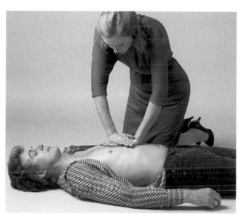

Make sure you keep your hand on the chest wall, pressing only on the line midway between the nipples. Apply the full weight of your body for an adult—use less pressure on a baby or child.

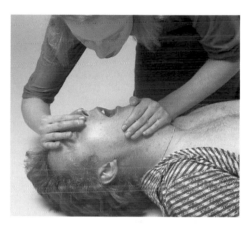

Mouth-to-mouth resuscitation has to be given simultaneously. If possible, someone else should do this. A breath should be blown in after every fifteenth heart compression.

the xiphoid. The palm of the hand should be placed on this point, and the palm of the other hand immediately on top of it. The movement of pressing down on the patient's chest should be rhythmic and regular, at a rate of 60 times a minute. The body's full weight must be applied if the patient is an adult, and this is most effectively done if the arms are kept straight at the elbows. Children and babies require a much lower pressure, and only one hand or a thumb should be used.

When one person is combining cardiac compression with expired air resuscitation, he or she should blow in two breaths during every 15 heart compressions, but no pause in the sequence of compressions should be allowed for a breath to be given. Even if two people are working together, one of them should still blow in one breath for every 15 compressions that the other gives. Although in adults the ideal rate is 60 beats per minute at an uninterrupted rhythm, in children this rate should be speeded up. Infants and children up to five years old should be squeezed at about 100 beats per minute, those between the ages of five and ten at about 80 beats per minute. Older children should receive compressions at 60 beats per minute (as for adults).

The carotid pulse in the neck should be checked every two minutes to see if the pulse has returned. Once this occurs, cardiac compression can be stopped. Usually, the heartbeat will return within a few minutes. The patient will begin to breathe again, the skin's gray hue will disappear, and the dilated pupils will return to normal.

Dangers

There is no danger of starting up an irregular heartbeat or stopping the heart, but overenthusiastic chest compression may damage soft organs lying under the lower parts of the ribs, resulting in a ruptured liver, stomach, or spleen. Ribs may get broken, but this is a risk worth taking. Generally, if heart compression is done properly, adequate force and squeezing action should depress the sternum by only 1 to 2 inches (2.5 to 5 cm) and no damage will be done.

See also: **Blood; Breathing; Circulatory system; Drug abuse; Electrocardiogram; Hemorrhage; Oxygen; Pulmonary disorders; Resuscitation; Unconsciousness**

Carpal tunnel syndrome

Our hands are extremely sensitive and capable of a wide range of movements, but in carpal tunnel syndrome both sensitivity and movement are reduced as the flow of messages between the brain and the hands is restricted.

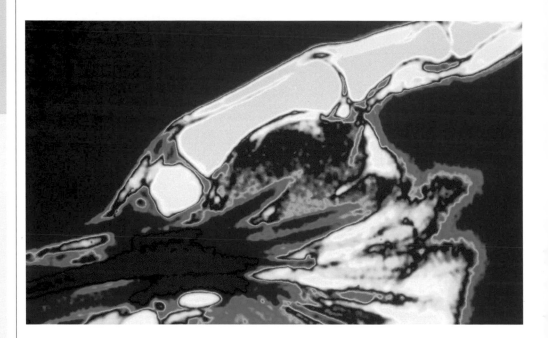

▲ *This color magnetic resonance imaging (MRI) scan shows the hand of a person with carpal tunnel syndrome. The bones of the thumb (top) show white; the tendons and ligaments (left) show blue and pink. The carpal tunnel lies under these ligaments.*

The hands, especially the surfaces of the fingertips, are among the most sensitive parts of the human body. They are also extremely powerful and versatile, being capable of performing a wide range of intricate movements. Some nerves carry signals between the brain and the hands, controlling how the hands move and feel. If one of these nerves—the median nerve—is pinched as it passes through the wrist, the condition known as carpal tunnel syndrome develops.

Structure of the hand and wrist

The hands and wrists are made up of a number of small bones and joints (see Hand; Wrist). Each hand contains five bones in the palm, known as the metacarpals. One end of four of these bones is joined to a finger, which consists of three bones, or phalanges, with a joint between each. The end of the fifth metacarpal bone is joined to the thumb, with two phalanges and a single joint. The hands are joined to the bones of the forearms— the radius and the ulna—by the wrists. Each wrist is made up of eight separate bones called carpals. They are arranged in two rows and are bound together by about 20 ligaments and tendons. The wrist bone that is visible as a bump under the surface of the skin is one of the carpals. The tendons and the median nerve that supply the hand are enclosed in a tough membrane that prevents the tendons from stretching the skin when the hand is flexed (pulled forward). The wrist bones above and the membrane below form a tunnel called the carpal tunnel. Because this passageway is narrow and rigid, if the tissues inside it swell for any reason, they crush the nerve and tendons, pressing them against the bones.

Symptoms and causes

Carpal tunnel syndrome may affect one or both hands and usually begins with a sensation of numbness, especially in the thumb and the next two and a half fingers, as the median nerve is crushed. This is followed by pins and needles, the unpleasant, tingling feeling that occurs as the crushed nerve recovers and sensation returns to the hand and fingers. The forearm and the thumb are often also very painful. The pain is generally worse at night and may be bad enough to wake a person from a deep sleep. The reason why the condition should be more painful at night is not clear, but if this is the case, hanging the hand over the side of the bed and rubbing or shaking it can sometimes help to lessen the pain. The symptoms may be brought on by overusing the hands for intricate work, such as sewing or knitting, or by activities that involve strenuous or repeated use of the wrists. Playing tennis or squash can exacerbate the symptoms.

Other conditions

Carpal tunnel syndrome can also be caused by other medical conditions, including diabetes, rheumatoid arthritis, and an underactive thyroid gland. An individual may also develop the syndrome if he or she fractures the wrist and causes some internal damage that puts pressure on the median nerve. Some women also find that they develop the syndrome during pregnancy, but in this case it nearly always disappears shortly after the birth, when the swelling that caused it also disappears.

In some people the condition is particularly severe and is likely to cause permanent numbness and weakness of the thumb and involve one or more of the fingers.

▼ *Sports that involve strenuous or repeated use of the wrists can sometimes lead to carpal tunnel syndrome. In such cases stopping the activity may be necessary.*

Treatment

Most people who suffer from carpal tunnel syndrome do not need any specific treatment. The symptoms gradually ease of their own accord as soon as the swelling or pressure affecting the nerve is reduced: for example, by stopping a strenuous or repetitive activity. Wearing a splint on the affected wrist at night may help to ease the pain. It is advisable not to take up a similar form of activity, even when the symptoms have disappeared, without consulting a doctor.

In some cases the doctor may advise treatment with drugs. Diuretic drugs will reduce the amount of fluid in the swollen tissues, and an injection of an anti-inflammatory drug into the wrist joint can help to reduce inflammation; both treatments will reduce the pressure on the nerve. In individuals whose carpal tunnel syndrome is caused by diabetes, rheumatoid arthritis, or an underactive thyroid gland, control of these diseases can alleviate carpal tunnel syndrome. If the syndrome is particularly persistent, or if it recurs at frequent intervals or causes severe pain, it can be permanently cured by surgery to reduce the pressure on the nerve. This may involve cutting through the tough membrane to create more space for the nerve. Sometimes some of the swollen or damaged tissue is removed at the same time as the nerve.

The surgical procedure is usually highly successful, and the symptoms disappear at once. It leaves a small scar on the inside of the wrist that fades to become insignificant.

See also: **Diabetes; Numbness; Inflammation; Repetitive strain injury; Rheumatoid arthritis; Sports injury; Surgery; Tendons**

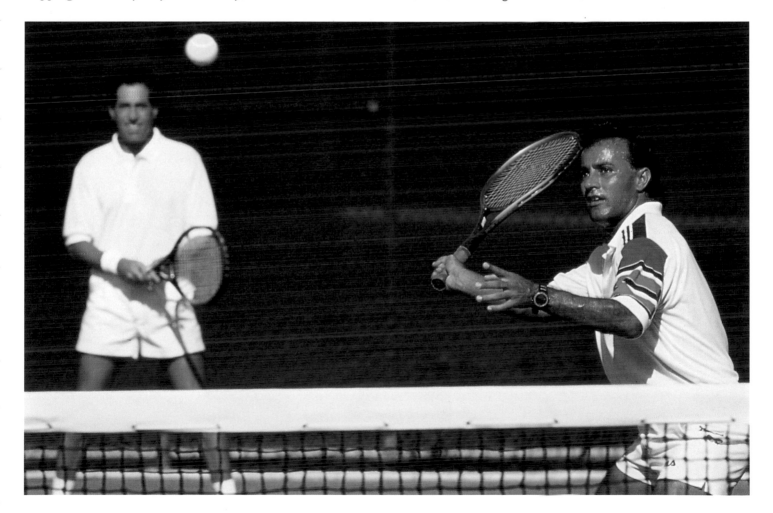

Cartilage

Questions and Answers

My toddler is always falling over but has never broken any bones. Is she just lucky?

A child's skeleton contains a great deal of cartilage. This is much tougher and more flexible than true bone and has more shock-absorbing power; that is why your daughter can take countless falls without breaking any bones. Falling is also less damaging to the young because they weigh less than adults. Also, the younger they are, the less fear they have, and therefore they do not get tense as they feel themselves falling. This is why you may occasionally hear of babies falling several stories out of buildings and literally bouncing.

My brother had the cartilage taken out of his knee. How can he manage without it?

The cartilage of the knee is part of the movement system of the joint. If the cartilage is removed, the joint is less efficient for a while, but then the muscles learn to compensate for the missing cartilage.

I am 63, and I recently discovered that I am 2 in. (5 cm) shorter now than when I was a girl. Why?

As the body ages, not only do the bones in the vertebral column get smaller, but the disks of cartilage between them get thinner and harder. This makes the disks shrink in size; with bone shrinkage, this makes you shorter.

My joints click loudly whenever I bend down. What is wrong?

Your bones click because the movement releases a vacuum in the joint. A high-pitched clicking sound is nothing to worry about, but if the sound gets deeper and there is pain, see your doctor.

The different types of cartilage form a vital part of the body's framework. Among its many functions, it surrounds the bronchial tubes, supports the nose and ears, and lines bones and joints.

Cartilage, or gristle, is a smooth, tough, but flexible part of the body's skeletal system. In adults it is mainly found in joints and covering the ends of bones, but it forms the complete skeleton of a developing fetus (see Skeleton). True bone forms in it. Cartilage that is subject to a great deal of wear and tear may cause problems, particularly in the spine and knees.

Nearly all the bones in the body begin as rods of cartilage, which gradually become hardened by deposits of calcium and other minerals. This process, which is called ossification, begins before birth, in the third or fourth month of fetal development.

Ossification is not fully complete until about the age of 21, since the cartilage not only forms the foundation for bone formation but also allows the bones to grow. In adults, however, cartilage remains at strategic points in the skeleton, where its toughness, smoothness, and flexibility are most needed.

THE DIFFERENT TYPES OF CARTILAGE

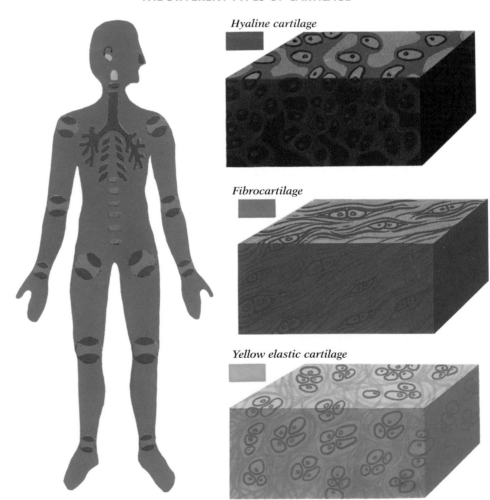

Hyaline cartilage

Fibrocartilage

Yellow elastic cartilage

▲ *Hyaline cartilage lines bones in joints and forms the respiratory tract. Fibrocartilage acts as a shock absorber in the backbone and other joints. Elastic cartilage is extremely flexible and forms the outer ear and the epiglottis in the throat.*

Structure

The structure of cartilage is not the same throughout the skeleton. Its makeup varies according to the specific job it has to do. All cartilage is composed of a groundwork, or matrix, in which there are embedded cells plus fibers made up of substances called collagen and elastin. The consistency of the fibers varies according to the type of cartilage, but all cartilage is alike in that it contains no blood vessels. Instead, it is nourished by nutrients that diffuse through the covering (perichondrium) of the cartilage, and lubricated by synovial fluid, which is made by membranes lining the joints (see Joints). According to its different properties, cartilage is known as hyaline cartilage, fibrocartilage, and elastic cartilage.

Types of cartilage

Hyaline cartilage is a bluish white, translucent tissue and, of the three types, has the fewest cells and fibers. What fibers there are all consist of collagen. This cartilage forms the fetal skeleton and is capable of the immense amount of growth that allows a baby to grow from about 18 inches (45 cm) into a person up to 6 feet (1.8 m) tall or more. After growth is complete, hyaline cartilage remains in a very thin layer, only 0.039 inch (1 mm) across, on the surface of the ends of the bones in the joints.

Hyaline cartilage is also found in the respiratory tract, where it forms the end of the nose and the stiff but flexible rings surrounding the windpipe and the larger tubes (bronchi) leading to the lungs. At the end of the ribs, bars of hyaline cartilage form the connections between the ribs and the breastbone and play their part in enabling the chest to expand and contract during breathing.

In the larynx, or voice box, hyaline cartilage not only helps to support the structure but is also involved in the production of the voice. As it moves, it controls the amount of air passing through the larynx, and therefore the pitch of the note that is emitted.

The second type, fibrocartilage, is composed of many bundles of the tough substance collagen, which makes it both resilient and able to withstand compression. Both these qualities are essential at the site in which fibrocartilage is most plentiful: between the bones of the vertebral column. In the spine each bone or vertebra is separated from its neighbor by a disk of fibrocartilage. The disks cushion the spine against jarring and help the human frame to remain upright. Each disk is made up of an outer coating of fibrocartilage that surrounds a thick, syrupy fluid. The cartilaginous part of the disk, which has a lubricated surface, prevents the bones from being worn away during movement, and the fluid acts as a sort of natural shock absorber. Fibrocartilage also forms a tough connection between bones and ligaments; in the hip girdle it joins the two parts of the hips together at the symphysis pubis joint (see Ligaments). In women this cartilage is particularly important because it is softened by the hormones of pregnancy to let the baby's head pass through.

The third type of cartilage is known as elastic cartilage. It is made up of fibers of elastin, with collagen. The elastin fibers give elastic cartilage a distinctive yellow color. Strong but supple, elastic cartilage forms the flap of tissue called the epiglottis, which snaps down over the entrance to the airway as food is swallowed.

Elastic cartilage also makes up the springy part of the outer ear and supports the walls of the canal leading to the middle ear and the eustachian tubes that link each ear with the back of the throat. Along with hyaline cartilage, elastic cartilage forms part of the supporting and voice-producing areas of the larynx.

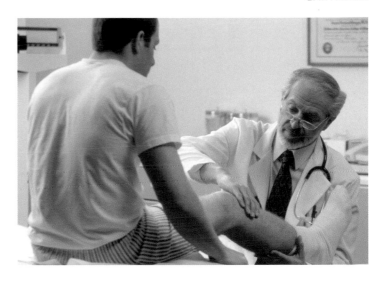

▲ *Torn cartilage in the knee is a common problem for professional soccer players.*

Problems and treatment

The cartilage that has to withstand constant pressure in the knees and vertebral column is the most vulnerable. The knee joint contains a pair of cartilage structures shaped like half moons, and they are most likely to be damaged by strenuous sports, particularly sports in which the knee joint is frequently twisted. If one or both half-moons become torn, and their frayed ends get caught between the surface of the joint, the knee will lock or give way. In such injuries, which are 20 times more common in men and are a notorious problem for soccer players, the knee should be firmly bandaged. In severe cases a splint may be needed behind the knee. The doctor may try to manipulate the joint to move the torn ends of the cartilage away from the joint surface, and to remove some of the excess fluid that accumulates around the site of the injury. However, the only way to cure the complaint completely is by surgical removal of the offending cartilage. The surgeon makes an incision from the bony lump at the side of the knee to the base of the knee joint and takes out the cartilage. After surgery it is important to get the knee moving as soon as possible, and physiotherapy should be given.

A slipped disk is another common cartilage problem. Strain or sudden twisting movements can tear the disks of cartilage between the vertebrae of the spine, making the pulpy center protrude and pushing the whole disk out of shape. The protrusion can press on nerves, causing pain in the back and possibly in the buttocks, thighs, and one leg. Rest in bed used to be recommended, but now doctors may recommend gentle exercise, traction, manipulation, or the wearing of a corsetlike belt. If none of these is successful in curing the trouble, surgery may be required.

In old age the joints become stiffer as the cartilage covering the ends of the bones loses its smoothness. This is quite normal, but in a condition called osteoarthritis, the cartilage and parts of the underlying bone degenerate. Osteoarthritis is not only a disease of old age; it can affect athletes and people who put excess strain on their joints by being overweight. Analgesics should relieve the pain, and physiotherapy and heat treatment will ease the joints.

See also: Bones; Joint replacement; Sports injury

Cataracts

Questions and Answers

My doctor says I have to wait for my cataract to "mature" before it is removed. What does this mean?

This simply means the cataract has to develop to such a degree that surgery is necessary.
    A cataract can be removed at any stage, but it should not be removed unless vision will significantly improve after surgery. At the moment your eyesight has probably not deteriorated sufficiently to require surgery.

My uncle had cataracts removed. Can I avoid getting them?

Don't worry; they are not hereditary or contagious. Cataracts are usually a result of advancing age, but ultraviolet light may cause cataracts, so wear sunglasses on bright days.

I had successful cataract surgery. Why is my vision still so poor?

The power of the lens implant may not exactly correct your vision for distance, and glasses may be needed. Even if the lens is correct for distance, you will still require reading glasses for sharp near vision. Current lens implants are of fixed focus. Surgery may have changed the shape of your cornea, causing astigmatism, which can be corrected by glasses. A more unfortunate possibility is that you may have retinal disease such as macular degeneration.

How can I tell whether someone has a cataract?

The opacity is in the internal lens behind the iris. If it is at the back of the lens, the eye may look normal, but if the opacity is dense and involves the front of the lens, a whitish pupil is seen. A scar from injury or disease may also cause a milky film over the eye.

Cataracts are a common condition of the lens of the eye. If left untreated they can lead to severe visual impairment, but modern surgical techniques are very effective in restoring good vision.

The term "cataract" dates from many centuries ago, when the appearance of whiteness was attributed by physicians to a kind of miniature waterfall descending from the brain to the eye. The lens is a minor focusing part of the eye, situated in a capsule immediately behind the pupil; the bulk of the work is done by the cornea, which is itself a fixed-focus lens (see Eyes and Eyesight). A cataract—a white opacity—can form in the lens, dimming vision until only light and dark can be seen. Eventually the cataract reaches a "mature" state and, if not surgically treated, it can give rise to secondary effects that, in some cases, can damage the eye. Such complications are uncommon, however, and it is rare for cataracts to lead to a permanent loss of vision.

Causes

The most common cause of cataracts is old age, in which case the cataracts mostly affect the center of the lens first. Blindness is delayed for many years until eventually the whole lens is affected. Some cataracts are congenital—that is, people are born with them. Within the first few months of human fetal development, the cells of many organs, including the eye, can suffer injury from infections or drugs that can enter the mother's blood system during pregnancy. The most serious maternal infection of early pregnancy that can cause congenital cataracts is rubella. This can also cause congenital heart disease and other serious misfortunes. All young girls should be protected by rubella vaccination before there is a risk of pregnancy (see Rubella).
    Other, less severe, congenital cataracts consist only of a light filming of the eye that resembles powder throughout the substance of the lens. Such cataracts rarely require any treatment at all, and vision is likely to remain good.

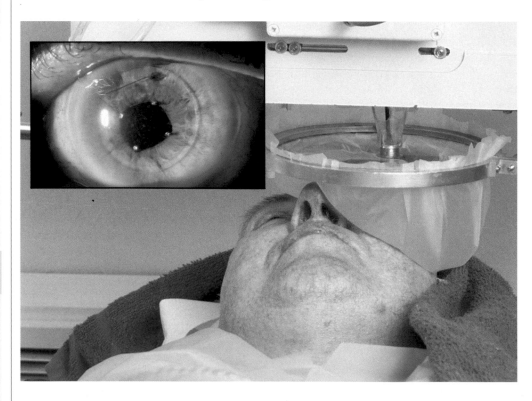

▲ *Cataracts can be removed by ultrasound. Very small incisions are made in the eye, and the cataract is washed out—the water bath is shown above.*

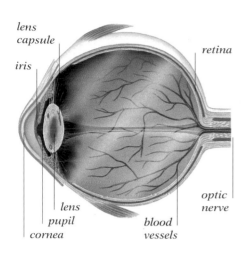

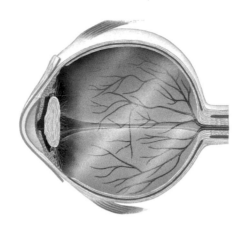

▲ *Section of an eye with a cataract. When a cataract affects only the center of the lens, dilation of the pupil with drops enables light to enter at the edges of the lens.*

▲ *One surgical method of removing a cataract —the extracapsular—involves removing the fibers of which the lens is formed, while leaving the lens capsule itself in place.*

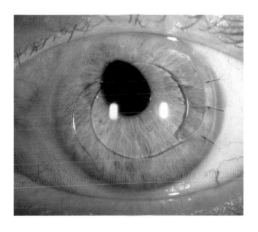

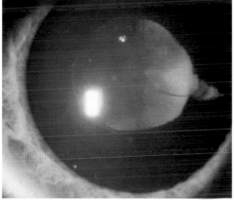

▲ *The most common way of getting rid of a cataract is to remove all opaque lens matter from the capsule of the lens, and to replace it with a tiny plastic lens, held in place by springy plastic loops.*

▲ *This close-up of an eye shows a congenital cataract—a condition that is relatively rare. It can be caused by an infection or by a drug in the mother's system during pregnancy.*

Diabetes is a rare cause of cataracts, but long-term diabetics often develop age-related cataracts at an earlier age than nondiabetics—sometimes up to 10 years earlier. In the early stages of diabetes, usually in adolescence, the sudden changes in blood-sugar levels can cause dense cataracts that come on in a matter of days. This is rare, and full vision is restored by simple surgery. A genetic disorder, galactosemia, causes high blood levels of an abnormal sugar and can cause cataracts in babies. This can be prevented by giving a galactose-free diet. Cataracts can form for other reasons, too. A high concentration of drugs in the blood can have a toxic effect on the lens; and steroid drugs, taken by mouth, as eyedrops, or by injection, may induce cataracts if given over a long period. Exposure to electromagnetic, cosmic, microwave, or infrared radiation can have a similar effect. Cataracts can be formed as a result of accidents and industrial and recreational injuries. A blow to the eye will sometimes cause a cataract to develop, usually within

hours. A miniscule injury from a needle, thorn, or metal foreign body, if it involves the lens capsule or the lens itself, can lead to a similar problem—immediately or sometimes many years afterward.

Symptoms

The most obvious symptom of cataracts is a loss of distinct vision, and sometimes the inability to see in bright light. Cataracts commonly alter the perception of colors so that everything seen may have a yellowish, or even reddish, tinge. This is often inapparent if both eyes are equally affected, but if the cataract is one-sided for a time, the effect may be more obvious when the vision in the two eyes is compared. After surgery, patients will commonly express surprise at the vividness of the color of blue objects or of the sky. This phenomenon is due to the greater absorption of light of long wavelength by the cataract. Another symptom of maturing cataracts, with increasing density of the lens substance, is progressive short sight. This is called index myopia, and it is due to greater bending of light rays. The effect of index myopia is that a person who formerly required strong reading glasses may, for a time, be able to read without them. This advantage, however, is offset by poor distance vision, as is the case with all shortsighted people. Index myopia usually progresses fairly rapidly, and if glasses are obtained for distance vision, they are not likely to be suitable for more than a few months.

As the cataract matures, near vision is lost and finally only light and dark can be distinguished. Usually one eye is affected before the other, but nearly always both will show signs of developing cataracts, and if treatment is not given, blindness may occur. The term "blindness" is used here to imply loss of useful vision. A cataract does not cause blindness in the sense of total absence of the perception of light (see Blindness and Braille). However dense, a cataract will always allow the passage of diffuse light. A person with cataracts who has no perception of light in the affected eye must have some other disorder, usually of the retina or optic nerve, that has caused his or her blindness. In such a case, vision cannot be restored by surgery, and operative treatment would be unwarranted.

Treatment

When cataracts affect only the center of the lens, drops containing drugs that dilate the pupil are helpful; they enable light to enter the eye at the outer edges of the lens. The majority of cataracts affect the entire lens, and the only effective treatment is surgery. There are three basic surgical methods, depending upon a person's age and the type of cataract present. In children and young people, the lens

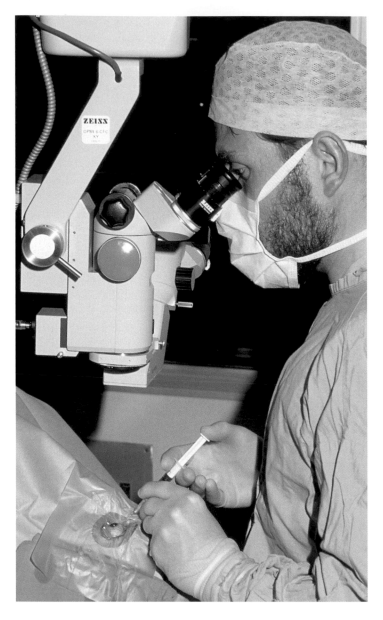

◀ *A surgeon scans a microscope suspended over the patient while performing the delicate surgery required to remove a cataract from the patient's eye.*

can be used in the treatment of any age group. The advantage of this method is that only small incisions into the eye are necessary. The disadvantage is that a second operation is sometimes necessary later to produce better vision.

The third and most common type of operation, used in patients over the age of 20, also involves the removal of all lens matter within the lens capsule. In this method the eye is opened, and the front capsule of the lens is carefully cut away. The opaque nucleus of the lens is gently squeezed out of the capsule and removed from the eye. All residual opaque lens matter is now scrupulously removed by washing and suction. If any lens matter is left, vision will be impaired. The inside surface of the back capsule is also carefully cleared of lens matter by a delicate polishing technique. A tiny plastic lens of predetermined power and fitted with supporting loops is now inserted into the empty capsule, where it is automatically centered by the springy loops. The incision in the cornea is closed using a continuous zigzag stitch, using material finer than a human hair. Healing of the incision takes about a month, and it is usually unnecessary to remove the stitch. The results of this operation, which is the routine procedure for adult cataracts, are usually excellent. Assuming that the eye is otherwise healthy, there is no reason why full vision should not be restored.

Correction of vision

Although every effort is made to select the correct lens power, this is not always possible in practice. The normal optical methods of determining the power of the eye and the appropriate correction that will be required when the lens is removed cannot always be used before surgery takes place. In an attempt to achieve accuracy, it is common to measure the internal axial length of the eyeball by means of an ultrasonic beam, produced by a specialized ophthalmic machine. The curvature of the cornea is also usually determined by another machine, called a keratometer.

These data, together with prior information on the power of the glasses used before the cataract developed, will enable the surgeon to calculate the power of lens implant most likely to produce normal distance vision without glasses.

If this is achieved, regular reading glasses will then be needed for close work. Sometimes the outcome is a minor degree of short sight, so that reading is possible without glasses. In this case glasses will be needed for clear distance vision.

Outlook

A number of undetermined factors, including limitations in the accuracy of measurements, may, however, make either of these outcomes impossible. In addition, slight variations in the tension of the stitch used to close the operation incision may induce some degree of astigmatism in the cornea. (Astigmatism means that the corneal curvature is flatter than normal along one meridian.) In such cases a spectacle correction (glasses) may be needed, for both distance and near vision.

matter remains soft, even after a cataract has developed, and can be removed fairly easily by one of several possible techniques. The operation is done under general anesthesia, and drops are used to widen the pupil as fully as possible. The surgeon uses an operating microscope and very delicate instruments. Typically a tiny, oblique incision is made on either side of the cornea, and a sharp, hollow needle is passed through one of these and a fine, blunt tube through the other. A source of sterile salt solution, formulated to produce minimal irritation to the eye, is connected to the tube. The sharp needle is then used to perforate the front capsule of the lens, and as the solution is run into the eye to maintain its shape, the lens matter is sucked out through the sharp needle. This procedure is continued until the pupil is completely clear. No stitches are required. After the operation the eye will be grossly unfocused, and an optical correction will be required. In young people this is best provided in the form of contact lenses. Some surgeons will, however, insert plastic implants into the eye at the time of the operation.

The second method to remove a cataract is by ultrasound (phacoemulsification). This advanced procedure combines the opening of the lens capsule and the washing out of the cataract, and

See also: **Astigmatism; Congenital disorders; Cornea; Diabetes; Steroids**

Celiac disease

Celiac disease makes sufferers unable to tolerate gluten, a substance found in foods made from wheat, rye, barley, and oats. The condition is controlled by avoiding these foods.

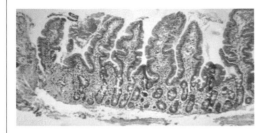

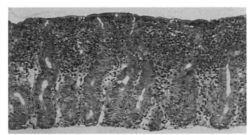

▲ *Microscopic views show the lining of the jejunum (part of the small intestine) when normal (top), and in a patient with celiac disease (above).*

Celiac (pronounced see-lee-ack) disease means disease of the belly, although the name is inaccurate because the complaint is a disorder of the lining of the intestine. Sufferers have an intolerance (a form of allergy) to gluten—a natural protein found in wheat and other cereals—and the disorder stops the body from absorbing fats, calcium, and other important nutrients from food (see Digestive System). No one knows why gluten damages the intestines of sufferers; this effect could be due to an allergy, to the lack of an enzyme that breaks down gluten, to an abnormality in the intestinal membrane, or to a combination of all these causes. Fortunately the disease is not common, affecting only one person in 500, but it is a permanent condition and sufferers need to follow a gluten-free diet carefully.

The main symptom of celiac disease is weight loss. Other symptoms include diarrhea; a puffed-up, painful stomach; and the passing of pulpy, foul-smelling feces full of undigested fat. The disease is dangerous only if it is not diagnosed; then, anemia and malnutrition can result.

Diagnosing the disease in babies is simple because the symptoms are obvious: they are sick and bloated and fail to put on any weight. Otherwise, tests for the disease are undertaken at gastroenterology clinics. The patient swallows a small capsule attached to a special tube, an X ray is taken, and then a sample of the intestinal lining is retrieved through the tube. In a healthy person the lining is covered with tiny fingerlike fronds called villi; in celiac sufferers these are destroyed.

The only effective treatment for celiac disease is a gluten-free diet. Once gluten is avoided, the villi grow back and the condition of the sufferer improves in time. Treatment is not a cure, however, and the villi will disappear if the person starts eating gluten again. Avoiding gluten is not always easy, but gluten-free products and alternatives are available.

A gluten-free diet

Avoid all foods made from, or containing, gluten. This includes anything containing wheat, rye, barley, or oats.

When in doubt, check the ingredients listed on the label.

Some gluten-free products carry a special symbol: a circle containing a crossed-out ear of wheat.

Use gluten-free varieties of the following foods:
  Baby foods (cereals, vegetables, fruits)
  Spaghetti
  Macaroni
  Semolina
  Cookies
  Flour
  Bread (bread mix, canned white or
    brown bread)
  Baking powder
  Cakes
  Crackers
  Topping and cookie mixes
  Bedtime drinks
  Soup mixes
  Soy bran

See also: Anemia; Malnutrition; X rays

Cells and chromosomes

Do the number of cells in a child's body increase as he or she grows?

Yes. A person has millions more cells as an adult than at birth, although the increase is not evenly distributed throughout the body. The number of cells in the brain, for example, increases much less as the body develops than the number in the bones, skin, and muscles.

I have heard that certain creams can revitalize my cells. Will they really stop the aging process?

No. There are no preparations that can stop the gradual deterioration and replacement of cells or reverse the changes that take place in cells as they age.

I have read that nuclear radiation can cause birth abnormalities. Why?

Nuclear radiation can kill cells, and it can produce permanent changes called mutations in the chromosomes—the parts of the cell that carry hereditary instructions. If these changes affect the chromosomes of the eggs or sperm, which are brought together at the moment of fertilization to produce a new individual, then an abnormal baby can result. If the baby survives into adulthood, he or she could well pass on the abnormality to future generations.

My twin girls are identical. Are their cells the same, and if so, why?

Identical twins are born when an egg from the mother splits in two after it has been fertilized by a sperm from the father; thus the twins are always the same sex and always carry exactly the same genetic instructions. Scientists find identical twins fascinating because all the differences that exist between them must be due to environmental factors.

Every part of the body is composed of millions of microscopic cells. In the nucleus of each of these are strands of DNA, which contain the genetic instructions that determine the characteristics each person inherits.

The cells are the basic units of life, the microscopic building blocks from which the body is constructed. Within the cells are the lengths of DNA that contain the vast amount of information essential to the creation and maintenance of human life and an individual's personal characteristics. Every adult body contains more than 100 million cells, microscopic structures averaging only 0.00039 inch (0.01 mm) in diameter. No one cell can survive on its own outside the body unless it is cultured (artificially bred) in special conditions, but when grouped together into tissues, organs, and systems of the body, the cells work together in harmony to sustain life.

Types and structures

The body cells vary greatly in shape, size, and detailed structure according to the jobs they do. Muscle cells, for example, are long and thin and contain fibers that can contract and relax, allowing the body to move. Many nerve cells are also long and thin, but they transmit electrical impulses that compose the nerve messages. The hexagonal cells of the liver are equipped to carry out a multitude of chemical processes, doughnut-shaped red blood cells transport oxygen and carbon dioxide around the body, and spherical cells in the pancreas make and replace the hormone insulin.

Despite these variations, all body cells are constructed according to the same basic pattern. Around the outside of every cell is a boundary wall or cell membrane enclosing a jellylike substance, the cytoplasm. Embedded in the cytoplasm is the nucleus that houses the genetic instructions in the DNA. The cytoplasm, although between 70 and 85 percent water, is far from inactive. Many chemical reactions take place between substances dissolved in this water, and the cytoplasm also contains tiny structures called organelles, each with an important and specific task. The cell membrane also has a definite structure: it is porous, and it is rather like a sandwich of protein and fat, with the fat as the filling. As substances pass into or out of the cell, they are either dissolved in the fat or passed through the porous, semipermeable membrane.

Some cell membranes have hairlike projections called cilia. In the nose, for example, these trap dust particles. The hairs can also move in unison to waft substances along in a certain direction.

PARTS OF A CELL

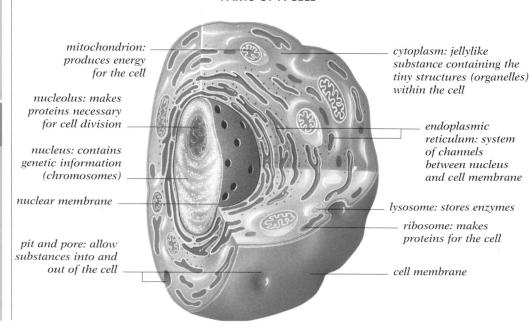

mitochondrion: produces energy for the cell

nucleolus: makes proteins necessary for cell division

nucleus: contains genetic information (chromosomes)

nuclear membrane

pit and pore: allow substances into and out of the cell

cytoplasm: jellylike substance containing the tiny structures (organelles) within the cell

endoplasmic reticulum: system of channels between nucleus and cell membrane

lysosome: stores enzymes

ribosome: makes proteins for the cell

cell membrane

DIFFERENT TYPES OF CELLS IN THE BODY

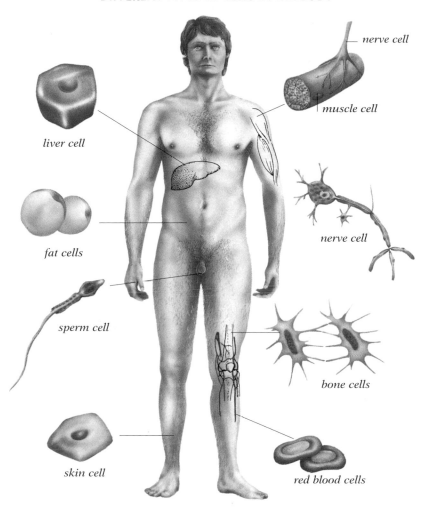

liver cell

nerve cell

muscle cell

fat cells

nerve cell

sperm cell

bone cells

skin cell

red blood cells

The cytoplasm of all cells contains microscopic, sausage-shaped organs called mitochondria, which convert oxygen and nutrients into the energy needed for all other cell actions. These powerhouses work through the action of enzymes—complex proteins that speed up chemical reactions. They are most numerous in the muscle cells, which need a vast amount of energy to carry out their work. Lysosomes—another type of microscopic organ in the cytoplasm—are sacs filled with enzymes that make it possible for the cell to use the nutrients with which it is supplied. The liver cells contain the greatest number of these. Further minute organs called the Golgi apparatus are necessary to package and store substances made by the cell, such as hormones, that are needed in other parts of the body.

Many cells also possess a network of tiny tubes that are thought to act as a kind of internal cell skeleton, and all of them contain a system of channels called the endoplasmic reticulum. Dotted along the reticulum are tiny spherical structures called ribosomes, which are responsible for controlling the construction of essential proteins. All cells need proteins for structural repairs and, in the form of enzymes, for cell chemistry and the manufacture of complex molecular structures such as hormones.

What is a chromosome?

Each nucleus is packed with information, coded in the form of a chemical called deoxyribonucleic acid (DNA), and organized into groups called genes. When cells are about to divide, the DNA coils up tightly to form chromosomes that are visible with an ordinary microscope. Every chromosome contains thousands of genes, each with enough information to produce one protein. This protein may have a small effect within the cell and on the appearance of the body, but equally it may make the difference between, for example, brown and blue eyes, straight and curly hair, normal and albino skin. The genes are responsible for every physical characteristic (see Genetics).

Apart from mature red blood cells, which lose their chromosomes in the final stages of their formation, and the eggs and sperm (the sex cells), which contain half the usual number of chromosomes, every body cell contains 46 chromosomes, arranged in 23 pairs. One of each pair comes from the mother and one from the father. The eggs and sperm have only half that number, so that when a sperm fertilizes an egg, the new individual has the correct number of chromosomes.

At the moment of fertilization, the genes start issuing instructions for the molding of a new human. The father's chromosomes are responsible for determining sex. These chromosomes are called X or Y, depending on their shape. In women both the chromosomes in the pair are X, but in men there is one X and one Y chromosome. If a sperm containing X fertilizes an egg, the baby will be a girl; but if a Y sperm fertilizes the egg, the baby will be a boy.

How a cell divides

In addition to being packed with information, the DNA of the chromosomes has the ability to reproduce itself; without this the cells could not duplicate themselves, nor could they pass on information from one generation to another. The process of cell division in which the cell duplicates itself is called mitosis; this is the type of division that occurs when a fertilized egg grows first into a baby and then into an adult, and when worn-out cells are replaced.

When the cell is not dividing, the chromosomes are not visible in the nucleus; but when the cell is about to divide, they become shorter and thicker and can be seen to split in half along their length. These double chromosomes then pull apart and move to opposite ends of the cell. Finally, the cytoplasm is halved and new walls form around the two new cells, each of which has the normal number of 46 chromosomes.

A huge number of cells die and are replaced by mitosis every day, but some cells are more efficient at this than others. Once formed, the cells of the brain and nerves are unable to replace themselves, but liver, skin, and blood cells are replaced several times a year.

Making cells with half the usual chromosome number, in order to determine inherited characteristics, involves a different type of cell division called meiosis. First the chromosomes become shorter and thicker (as in mitosis) and divide in two; at the moment of fertilization, the chromosomes pair up so that the one from the mother and the other from the father lie side by side. Next the chromosomes become tightly intertwined so that when they eventually pull apart, each new chromosome contains some of the mother's genes and some of the father's. After this the two new cells divide again so that each egg or sperm contains the 23 chromosomes it needs. The interchange of

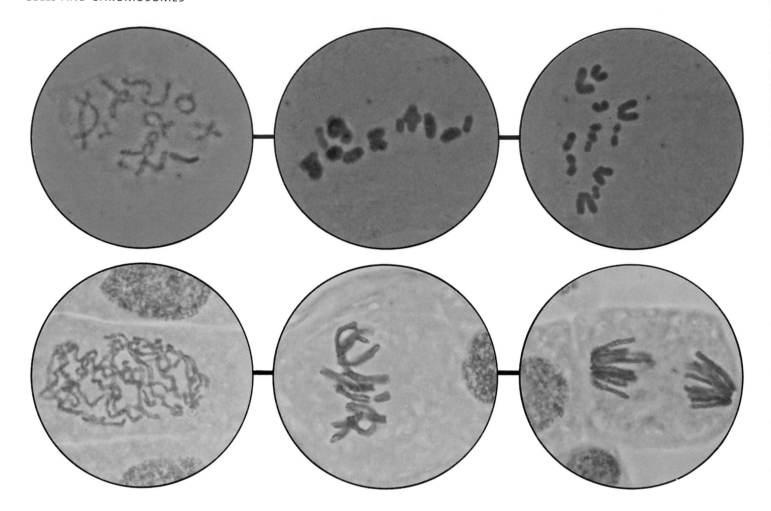

▲ ► *The main difference between the two methods of cell division are shown above, greatly enlarged. In meiosis (top sequence above), the chromosomes are duplicated and then pair up and intertwine, before pulling apart and dividing to produce sex cells containing half the genetic information needed to produce a human (the remaining half is supplied during fertilization). In mitosis (bottom sequence above), pairs of chromosomes separate, and each half divides into two identical parts. These arrange themselves so that when the respective parts move to opposite ends of the cell and the cell divides into two, each new cell will contain the genetic information necessary to replace or duplicate existing body cells. The illustration at right shows the structure of a chromosome in detail.*

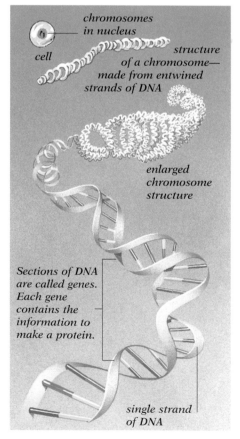

chromosomes in nucleus

cell

structure of a chromosome— made from entwined strands of DNA

enlarged chromosome structure

Sections of DNA are called genes. Each gene contains the information to make a protein.

single strand of DNA

genetic material during the process of meiosis explains why children do not look exactly like their parents and why each person, with the exception of identical twins, has a completely unique genetic makeup.

Problems

Considering the number of cells and the complexities of their structure and chemistry, it is surprising how little goes wrong during the average life, and how few babies are born with deformities. Apart from accidental damage and disease, things go wrong only when there is some abnormality of the chromosomes or of the genes they contain—so that faulty information is sent out to the cell—or if a cell is unable to respond to the messages it receives, although these are correct.

Sometimes entire chromosomes can be responsible for abnormalities. For example, children with Down syndrome are born with one extra chromosome, while extra sex chromosomes can cause abnormalities in sexual development. Many abnormalities at birth are caused by faulty genes. Other problems, such as muscular dystrophy, arise some time after birth, although these, too, are caused by faulty genes. Many aspects of cell life and action have yet to be clarified by science.

See also: **Enzymes; Hormones**

Cellular telephones

Questions and Answers

Why is it called a cellular phone?

The term "cellular" came about because the wireless system uses base stations, or broadcast towers, that divide a service area into many "cells" (ranges of service area). The phone calls are transferred from the closest tower or base station to the next as the mobile phone user travels from one cell to another.

Who invented the cellular phone?

The concept was first introduced by Bell Laboratories in 1947 from technology used in police cars. However, it was not until 1968 that the Federal Communications Commission (FCC), in charge of airwave regulation, agreed to provide enough radio-spectrum frequencies for a mobile phone service to be lucrative. In 1973 the first portable cellular phone was invented by Dr. Martin Cooper, a project manager at Motorola, and some of his colleagues.

There is concern about the risks of using cellular phones while driving. What is being done about this?

Federal legislation has been proposed that would let drivers make calls only if they use a hands-free device, such as an earpiece or a speakerphone. A Senate version of the law would let each state decide whether to allow this exemption to the ban on using phones while driving. If you must use a cellular phone on the road:

• Park or pull off the road. If you must answer a call, let the caller know you are driving and suspend the call.
• Make sure your phone is easy to see and reach so you don't have to take your eyes off the road.
• Get to know your phone's features to prevent fumbling.
• Use hands-free devices.
• Avoid stressful or emotional calls.
• Avoid calls while driving in hazardous conditions.

The increasing use of cellular telephones has given rise to concern over the risk that the electromagnetic radio-frequency radiation emitted by these phones may cause serious harm to people's health.

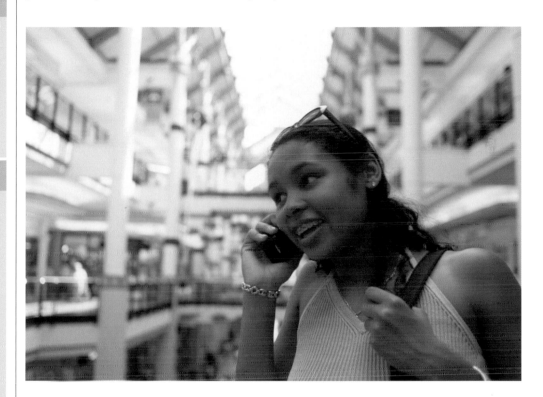

▲ *Research is currently being done to establish any links between cellular phones and cancers of the head and neck. Although no serious dangers to health have yet been established, children who use cellular phones may be at higher risk because their skulls and nervous systems are not fully developed. They should therefore take the precaution of using cellular phones only for short calls and only when necessary.*

In the early 21st century, the use of mobile phones soared, leading to fears that the potential risks of overuse had not been fully investigated. Most bodies, however, largely agree that further research is needed and that, as a precaution, children should limit their use of mobile phones and, when possible, send text messages instead. Children are frequent users of cellular phones, and because their nervous system is not fully developed and their skull is not fully mature, there is a possibility that they are more at risk than adults.

Research studies

It is predicted that there will be about 1.6 billion mobile phone users worldwide by the year 2005. Because of the massive numbers involved, even small numbers of people who might be adversely affected could have enormous implications for public health. Therefore any health risks must be established as soon as possible to avert a crisis. Studies to ascertain the risks are ongoing, but so far none has come to any definite conclusions.

The World Health Organization International Agency for Research on Cancer does not have any evidence that radiation emitted from cellphones is a health risk; however, it is continuing its investigations in 10 countries to establish whether there are links between head and neck cancers and the use of mobile phones (see Cancer). The U.N. Health Agency is also looking at whether radiation from cell phones causes an increase in these cancers, but says that in the meantime there is no need to introduce safety legislation. The Food and Drug Agency (FDA) plans

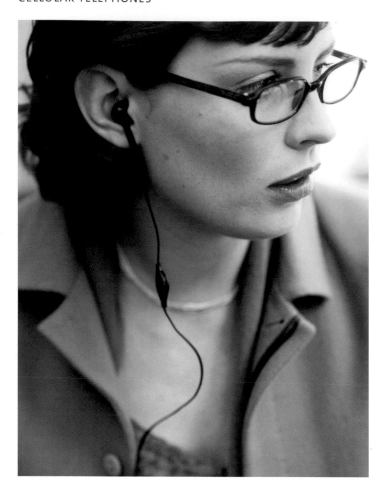

▲ *Headsets are recommended when using cellular phones because they allow for the phone to be held away from the head and neck, where the radiation emitted has less effect.*

to continue carrying out studies on safety aspects, although there have been no major research findings connecting mobile phones and illness. Many scientists believe that because the radiation from cellular phones is somewhere between the level of radiation emitted by microwave ovens and the level emitted by televisions, it is highly unlikely that cellular phones could be a risk to health.

Finnish study

A scientist for Finland's radiation and nuclear safety authority, Professor Darius Leszczynski, claims that radiation from cellular phones could weaken the cells in the blood-brain barrier, which is the layer of cells in the capillaries around the brain that protect the brain from toxins and microorganisms in the bloodstream (see Blood-Brain Barrier). During laboratory tests using human brain cells, he discovered that a critical protein was affected by radiation. Professor Leszczynski was not worried by his findings, but he felt that caution dictates the need for more research.

How cellular phones work

Cellular phones, or wireless phones, are handheld phones that have built-in antennas. They work like two-way radios; when someone sends a call, he or she talks into a cellular phone, which picks up the voice and converts it to radiofrequency energy in the form of radio waves. The radio waves travel to any nearby receiver at a base

station, which then sends the call through the telephone network until it reaches the person being called.

When a call is received on a cellular phone, the message goes through the telephone network to a base station near the recipient's phone. Radio waves are sent out from the base station to a receiver in the recipient's phone, where the signals are converted into the sound of a voice.

Regulation of cellular telephones

The Federal Communications Commission (FCC) and the FDA both monitor cellular phones. The FCC places limits on radiation emission from mobile phones and is responsible for ensuring that cellular phones adhere to safety guidelines governing radiofrequency energy. The FDA regulates the health effects of cellular phones to make sure that the radiation given off does not pose an unacceptable risk. If a cellular phone emits dangerous levels of energy, both agencies have the power to take action.

The FCC gets its authority to act on this issue from the National Environmental Policy Act of 1969 and the Telecommunications Act of 1996. The FDA is authorized by the Federal Food, Drug, and Cosmetic Act of 1968, which was originally the Radiation Control for Health and Safety Act.

Both the FCC and the FDA liaise with other agencies about radiofrequency radiation. These include the Occupational Health and Safety Administration, the Environmental Protection Agency, the National Institute for Occupational Safety and Health, and the National Telecommunications and Information Administration.

Research collaboration

The FDA is collaborating with the Cellular Telecommunications Industry Association (CTIA) on research into the safety of cellular phones. The research will be conducted by third parties in the interests of objectivity. It is estimated that the research will be complete in late 2005.

Health risks versus harm to the industry

Cellular technology has proved beneficial to emergency services, and to the exchange of information, and the public has become increasingly dependent on cellular services. Until there is any certain scientific proof of risk, responses from public protection agencies seek to avoid unnecessary harm to the cellular telecommunications industry, which at present offers a useful product.

Protective measures

To protect themselves, cellular phone users can make shorter calls, use a headset, and hold the device away from the body. In collaboration with the U.S. military, American scientists have developed a device that may quash worries about radiation from mobile phones. The device is the BioChip—a tiny microchip that is fitted to the battery in a cellular phone. The BioChip emits a weak electromagnetic impulse that is similar to a natural impulse to which brain cells are accustomed and prevents them from picking up the rhythm from the phone signal. This research was carried out because the U.S. Army was concerned about ill effects on soldiers from the radio telephones in their helmets.

See also: **Brain; Head and head injuries; Neck; Nervous system; Protein**

Cerebral palsy

The word "spastic" has wrongly become a slang term for a clumsy, stupid person. In fact, spastic people have cerebral palsy, or spasticity—a disabling disease, but one that may well not affect the individual's intelligence.

Cerebral palsy, sometimes called Little's disease, is a broad medical term that covers a range of conditions, all resulting in some form of paralysis in early infancy because of imperfect development of, or damage to, the nerve centers in the brain. The damage occurs during pregnancy, at birth, or soon after. There are approximately 300,000 children with cerebral palsy in the United States, and the most common form is spasticity, or spastic paralysis. There is a widely held misconception that all spastic people are mentally handicapped, but this is not true. Some people with this condition may have brain damage that affects their learning abilities, but many are of average or above-average intelligence. The condition is nonprogressive.

Types and causes

There are three main types of cerebral palsy, each affecting a different area of the brain. Spasticity accounts for more than 80 percent of all cases, and in this condition the outer layer of the brain, the cortex, appears to have been damaged. The cortex deals with such functions as thought, movement, and sensation—all vitally important. In athetosis, damage is centered on the inner part of the brain in a particular group of nerve cells known as the basal ganglia. These cells are responsible for easy, graceful flowing movement. The third type of cerebral palsy, ataxia, results when the cerebellum (situated at the base of the brain) is affected. The cerebellum connects to the brain stem, which links the main part of the brain with the spinal cord, and it controls balance, posture, and coordination of bodily movements (see Ataxia).

The largest single cause of cerebral palsy is thought to be prolonged oxygen starvation at birth. This may occur during a difficult or prolonged labor, when the baby's delicate brain

Questions and Answers

Is it correct to say that people who have no control over their muscles and their movements are spastic?

No. The term spastic can be used to describe a part of the body that does not work properly—for example, someone with a spinal injury may have spastic legs—but it is not a general term for people with cerebral palsy, even though they often have spastic limbs. Other conditions that may cause some paralysis include cerebral hemorrhage, Parkinson's disease, spina bifida, and multiple sclerosis.

Why can't some people with cerebral palsy speak properly, and can anything be done to help?

Several factors can cause speech difficulties in people with cerebral palsy. First, the speech center of the brain may be damaged. Second, a lack of good muscle control makes it hard to regulate breathing and form words. Third, people who find it difficult to control their speech may become tense when they try to speak, and this exacerbates the problem.

Speech therapy can help greatly, but the best help can come from the listener. Embarrassment will not help, so try to remember that the person is thinking just as quickly as you, but that physical factors prevent him or her from speaking normally.

My sister's son has congenital spasticity. Does this mean that any child of mine will also have this condition?

Don't confuse "congenital" with genetic. Congenital means that the condition was present at birth or soon afterward; genetic suggests that some inherited factor caused the baby to be spastic. Only a few cases are caused by an inherited factor, and it is rare to find more than one person with cerebral palsy in the same family.

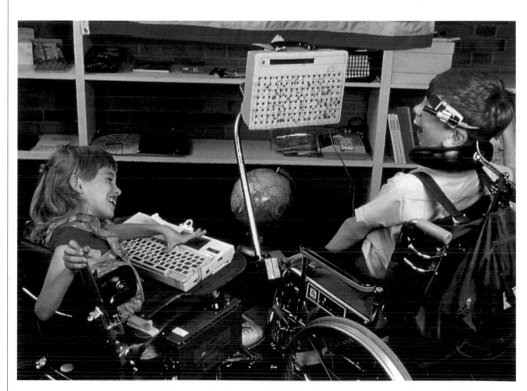

▲ *Voice synthesizers can help children with cerebral palsy who have severe speaking difficulties. The boy above controls his synthesizer using a laser attached to his headband.*

tissues, deprived of rich, oxygenated blood, can rapidly deteriorate. Certain illnesses and viruses during pregnancy can also affect the fetal brain; for example, rubella (German measles) in the early weeks of pregnancy is known to damage the fetus. Failure of the placenta to provide adequate nourishment can also cause difficulties, and some newborn babies may become brain-damaged after developing jaundice or as a result of infections such as meningitis and encephalitis. Injuries to the head can also result in cerebral palsy.

Symptoms

No two people with cerebral palsy have precisely the same degree of handicap. In some the brain damage is so mild that there is no apparent disability; in others the paralysis can affect all four limbs, speech, hearing, and vision; it may also cause mental handicap and epilepsy.

People with spasticity have general muscular stiffness, weakness, or paralysis in one or more limbs. They find it difficult to use or control the affected limb or limbs, and deformities can develop if treatment is not available. The paralysis can affect either side of the body (hemiplegia), the legs only (paraplegia), or all the limbs (diplegia, when the legs are mainly affected; and quadriplegia, when the legs and arms are equally involved). The paralysis can be either spastic, that is, stiff and rigid; or flaccid: limp and relaxed.

People with ataxia walk in an uncoordinated and awkward manner and usually have great difficulty in balancing. Those with athetosis are subject to involuntary, awkward movements and have difficulty controlling their limbs and the muscles in their faces and bodies.

Combinations of symptoms can mislead onlookers. For example, the involuntary, writhing movements and

▼ *This boy has athetosis, which makes it difficult for him to control his limbs and head. The facilities of a special school will help him fulfill his potential.*

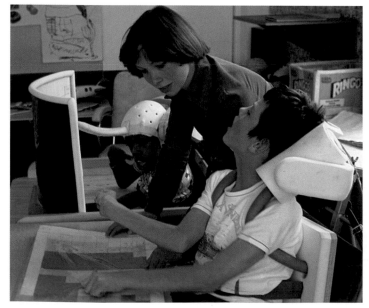

HOW CEREBRAL PALSY AFFECTS THE BRAIN

In spastic paralysis, damage to the cerebral cortex leads to uncontrolled movement, muscular weakness, and varying degrees of paralysis. Ataxia —difficulty in balance, posture, and coordination—results from damage to the cerebellum; and athetosis, characterized by involuntary movement, is caused when the basal ganglia are involved. In all these conditions sight, hearing, and speech may also be affected.

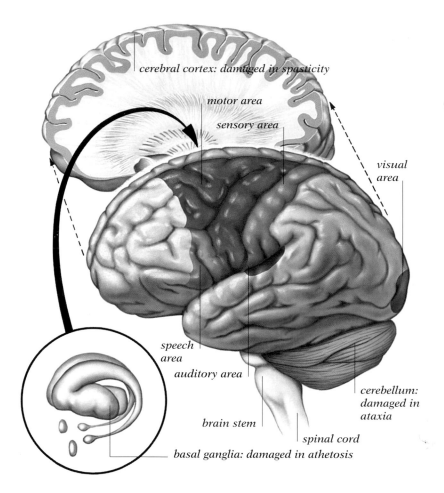

cerebral cortex: damaged in spasticity
motor area
sensory area
visual area
speech area
auditory area
cerebellum: damaged in ataxia
brain stem
spinal cord

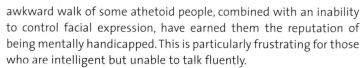
basal ganglia: damaged in athetosis

awkward walk of some athetoid people, combined with an inability to control facial expression, have earned them the reputation of being mentally handicapped. This is particularly frustrating for those who are intelligent but unable to talk fluently.

Hearing, sight, and speech may also be affected. If speech is badly slurred, the person may have difficulty in communicating, and when the hands are affected, learning can be difficult and slow. Some people with cerebral palsy also have epilepsy, and problems with spatial reasoning are not uncommon.

Treatment and outlook

There is no cure for cerebral palsy, but with therapy much improvement is possible. Physiotherapy can help movement in spastic muscles, and speech therapy is essential in assisting communication. As a result of technological developments, even the most severely handicapped can hope to live a reasonably fulfilled and satisfying life.

See also: **Encephalitis; Epilepsy; Jaundice; Meningitis; Rubella**

Cervix and cervical smears

Questions and Answers

Are cervical smear tests really necessary? I don't like the idea of them at all.

The incidence of cervix cancer in American women has fallen by 70 percent as a result of widespread use of the Pap smear test. Many thousands of lives have been saved by the test. In spite of this, over 13,000 American women get cervical cancer annually, and over 4,000 of them die from it each year. These women are mainly those who did not have Pap smear tests, perhaps simply because they didn't like the idea.

Isn't a Pap smear painful and embarrassing?

The doctor or the nurse is not embarrassed—it is just routine so there is no reason for you to be. You will not be able to see what is happening, so just relax, avoid squeezing, and the whole procedure should be painless.

What if my Pap smear test result indicates problems?

If you get what is called an abnormal result, don't panic. It may simply mean that the specimen was questionable and that the pathologist couldn't safely grade it as normal. It may have been taken too near the time of your period, it may have been badly preserved, or there may just be inflammatory changes, not cancer. Just make sure that you have a repeat test.

And if the result is truly abnormal?

Mildly abnormal cells call for a repeat test every three months or so. If there is a severe abnormality, you will have to have a biopsy of the cervix, a minor procedure in which a cone of cervix is removed for full microscopic examination. This procedure has saved many women from grave problems.

The cervix is the neck of the uterus, which remains closed until a woman gives birth. Cervical smears detect the presence of abnormal cells that can lead to cancer—if cancer is discovered early enough, treatment can provide a cure.

The cervix is the narrowed lower part, or neck, of the uterus. Although the uterus enlarges greatly during pregnancy, the cervix remains closed until the baby's head descends during childbirth and forces it open (see Uterus). The cervix is the site of various disorders, the most important of which is cancer.

Like the rest of the uterus, the cervix is largely muscular and is lined with a mucous membrane. It is almost cylindrical, about 1 inch (2.5 cm) long, and loosely connected to the bladder in front. The lower part of the cervix, which is somewhat conical and rounded, projects into the vagina so that there is a shallow cul-de-sac (or fornix) all around. This part of the cervix is covered with the same mucous membrane that lines the vagina and is readily accessible for examination. In the center of the vaginal part of the cervix is the tiny, circular external os (mouth), the mouth of the cervical canal that runs down the cervix from the cavity of the uterus.

Infections of the cervix

Cervical infections are fairly common and can cause inflammation (cervicitis). They are often sexually acquired and may be caused by herpes, chlamydia, gonorrhea, or syphilis (see Sexually Transmitted Diseases). All but the herpes virus respond well to treatment with antibiotics. Persistent (chronic) cervical infections can cause pelvic pain and backache, and there may be pain on intercourse. Infections with the human papillomavirus and herpes virus are believed to be important causal factors in cervical cancer. Because sexually promiscuous females have a higher chance of acquiring these viruses, they are more likely to develop cervical cancer. Some herpes strains, especially types 16 and 18, are classified as high-risk for cancer (see Herpes).

POSITION OF THE CERVIX

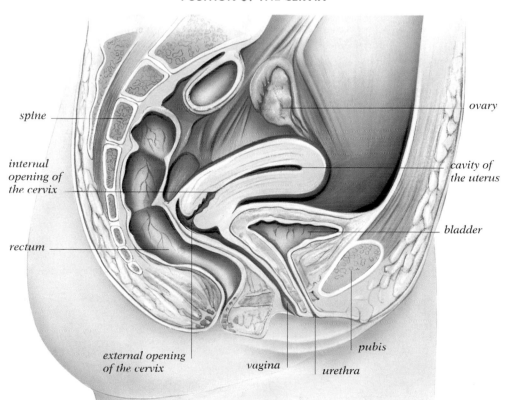

spine

internal opening of the cervix

rectum

external opening of the cervix

vagina

urethra

pubis

bladder

cavity of the uterus

ovary

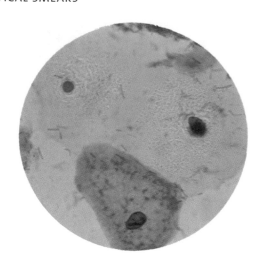

▶ *For a cervical smear a few cells are scraped off the lining of the cervix near the os. They are then placed on a glass slide, stained, and examined under a microscope to reveal any abnormalities. The cells to the right are normal.*

Cervical erosion

The term "cervical erosion" is a remnant from an earlier misinterpretation of the appearance commonly seen on direct visual examination of the cervix. It is inaccurate, because this appearance is not erosion or any other form of ulceration, nor is it an inflammation or the result of infection. Earlier gynecologists were convinced that cervical erosion was abnormal, and all kinds of symptoms were attributed to it. Many women underwent unnecessary treatment, especially cauterization with a hot probe.

The term refers to a conspicuous dark, raw-looking appearance of the outer part of the cervix, caused by an extension of the columnar epithelium (inner lining) of the canal of the cervix out onto the usually smooth and lighter-colored covering membrane of the vaginal part. The extension of this velvety red area onto the cervix is especially common during pregnancy, when the high levels of estrogen present cause it to expand and extend. Some contraceptive pills also produced well-marked "erosions" (see Oral Contraceptives).

Cervical erosion is seldom seen after a woman goes through menopause. This is a time when estrogen levels are lower, and any vaginal bleeding at this point must be taken more seriously (see Cancer; Estrogen).

Bleeding and discharge

Occasionally this extension of columnar epithelium, with its more profuse blood supply, leads to a slight, intermittent, bloodstained mucous discharge. It is a rule in gynecology that unexplained vaginal bleeding must never be ignored, so even bleeding from this cause should be investigated. If the cervical smear test gives a normal result in a pregnant woman, the condition can safely be ignored (see Gynecology; Pregnancy; Vagina).

Cervical incompetence

In some women the upper part of the narrow cervical canal is, for various reasons, abnormally open to just under 0.5 inch (1 cm) at the point at which it joins the cavity of the uterus. During pregnancy the internal pressure from the increasing volume of fluid surrounding the fetus (the amniotic fluid) tends to force this opening wider, so that the outlet of the uterus progressively expands. As a result, such women may repeatedly suffer the misfortune of painless, spontaneous miscarriages, usually around the fourth or fifth month of pregnancy. Miscarriage may also occur because the abnormal widening promotes premature rupture of the membranes.

This condition is known as cervical incompetence, and it is usually, although not always, a result of earlier damage to the cervix during delivery or previous surgery, such as a cone biopsy for suspected cancer, repeated dilatations and curettage, or an amputation of the cervix. When recognized, the condition is easily treated. At some time between the 12th week of pregnancy (when most spontaneous abortions have already occurred) and the 16th week, the cervix is reinforced with a single, strong, purse-string stitch of nonabsorbable material, such as nylon, sewn around it in an in-and-out manner. This procedure, known as the Shirodkar operation, keeps the cervix firmly closed until the baby can be safely delivered. The stitch is then cut and pulled out. This is a simple matter that takes only a few minutes.

Cervical smear

Cancer of the cervix is common. The cancer remains in the surface layer for years before invading the muscle. The smear test can detect it at this harmless stage. For this reason the cervical smear test should, ideally, be done on all females. The test can detect 90 percent of cell abnormalities, and treatment given during this preinvasive stage is simple, safe, and nearly always completely curative.

The cervical smear test, or Papanicolaou (Pap) smear (see Pap Smear), was instituted not by a gynecologist but by an American physiologist and microscopist, George Nicholas Papanicolaou (1883–1962). While investigating the reproductive cycle using vaginal smears, Papanicolaou recognized cancer cells and realized that this was an important way of diagnosing cervical cancer early. He then promoted the test among the medical profession and the general population.

The procedure

The Pap smear test is a simple, virtually painless, and highly reliable method of detecting cervical cancer in its earliest stages. The vagina is held open by a device called a speculum, and a shaped spatula is used in a rotary manner to gently scrape the area around the os for 360 degrees. The most important cells are those at the junction between the lining of the canal and the lining of the vaginal part of the cervix, known as the transformation zone, where cancer is most likely to start. The almost imperceptible smear of cells is put on a glass slide, fixed, stained, and then examined microscopically by an expert pathologist who has been trained to detect abnormalities in single cells. The whole technique is known as exfoliative cytology.

Suggested frequency

The test should be done regularly on all females, initially between the ages of 16 and 20 and every year thereafter. A three-year period between tests is the acceptable minimum requirement, except for those in whom the risk factors apply. These females should have the test at least once a year, or more often if abnormalities are found.

Pap smear tests should ideally be accompanied by microscopic examination of the cervix (colposcopy). This allows accurate localization of the abnormal surface tissue. The instrument used is a long-focus microscope with coaxial illumination that provides the gynecologist with an enlarged view of the vaginal part of the cervix.

Cancer of the cervix

Worldwide, cervical cancer is the most common female malignancy. Because of the Pap smear test, however, in the United States it now ranks only number eight in causes of death among women. This is a huge reduction and highlights the importance of the test.

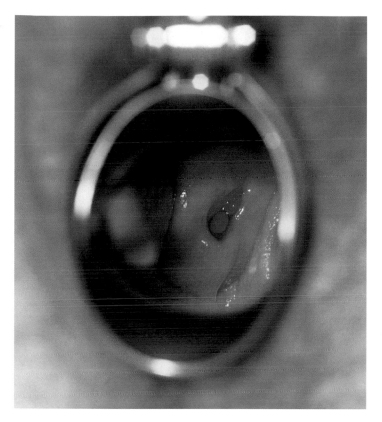

▲ *View of a cervical polyp, as seen through a cervical speculum. Polyps are benign growths that may occur on any mucous membrane; cervical polyps are removed if it is suspected that they may become malignant.*

Even so, the American Cancer Society states that, currently, some 12,900 new cases of invasive cervical cancer occur in the United States each year, causing 4,400 deaths. These deaths are particularly tragic when one considers how accessible the site of the cancer is and how easily it can be detected in the early stages if it is looked for. Laboratory tests to detect the types of human papillomaviruses (HPVs) that cause cancer are under development.

Another new test called the Hybrid Capture HPV Test may also prove useful in determining which women with abnormal Pap results should have a colposcopy. Vaccines against HPV are being developed and tested.

High-risk factors

Risk factors for cancer of the cervix include starting to have sexual intercourse at an early age, having many sexual partners, sexually-transmitted diseases, genital warts, repeated pregnancies, and cigarette smoking (see Intercourse).

As suggested, the sexual factors probably relate to the increased probability of infection with the human papilloma and herpes viruses. It is probably because of this that sexually promiscuous females are more likely to develop cervical cancer.

Research has shown that the DNA of human papillomavirus types 16 and 18 is found in 62 percent of women with cervical cancer, but in only 32 percent of women without cancer.

Other studies have shown that cervical cancer is more prevalent in those females who use drugs intravenously and in females who have had a positive HIV test.

Cervical intraepithelial neoplasia

Cancer of the cervix is preceded, for a number of years, by a recognizable and easily diagnosable preinvasive condition known as cervical intraepithelial neoplasia (CIN), or carcinoma-in-situ. The epithelium is the mucous membrane lining of the cervix, and neoplasia means a cancerous change in the cells. Intraepithelial means that these changes are still confined to the cells within the lining and thus have not invaded any other tissue. Cancer that remains at this stage is harmless, although potentially devastating. About 55,000 cases of CIN occur each year in the United States. Half of all cancers of the female reproductive system are in the cervix, and so early detection is essential for a course of treatment, which in many cases will provide a complete cure.

Symptoms

Cancer of the cervix often causes no symptoms until it has spread and may cause no symptoms at all before reaching an incurable stage. Sometimes there is bleeding between periods or following sexual intercourse, but there are no dramatic early signs.

Pain and general upset are rare until a late stage is reached and the cancer has spread to other sites. Such pain, which may be felt in the pelvis, buttocks, or lower back, often indicates that the disease is far advanced. It may imply that the cancer has spread widely into the pelvic or abdominal regions.

Involvement of the bladder and the rectum may cause blood in the urine or bleeding from the rectum. The moral is clear. Cancer of the cervix has to be looked for, and the best way to do this is by the Pap smear test.

Complications

Once the cancer has passed from the epithelium into the underlying cervical muscle, the treatment becomes more difficult. If the cancer is confined to the cervix, the choice rests between removing a cone of the cervical muscle and removing the whole uterus (simple hysterectomy). The former has a recurrence rate of about 5 percent; the latter, a zero recurrence rate (see Hysterectomy).

More extensive cervical cancer is difficult to treat successfully, and the choice rests between extensive surgery and radiotherapy. There is no universal agreement on which of these forms of treatment is best. Radiotherapy is widely used—this treatment is usually administered by means of a sealed container of radioactive material placed in the vault of the vagina and in the cavity of the uterus.

Outlook

The cure rate for cervical cancer depends on the extent of its spread at the time of diagnosis. If it has spread to the vagina and surrounding tissues, the cure rate drops sharply to about 50 percent.

Extensive spreading to the organs of the pelvis and remote spreading to other parts of the body has a very poor outlook. In only about 10 percent of such cases is the patient still alive five years later. When the condition is detected in its early stages by means of the Pap smear test, there is an excellent chance of cure and recovery for many women who suffer from this type of cancer.

> *See also:* **AIDS; Biopsy; Bladder and bladder problems; Cells and chromosomes; Genitals; Gonorrhea; Hormones; Pelvis; Radiotherapy; Syphilis**

Cesarean birth

I was so disappointed at not giving birth naturally that I cannot help feeling like a failure. I have been depressed and at times find it hard to feel affection for the baby. How can I get over this?

First, having a cesarean is not a failure on your part. It was a necessity beyond your control. Women who have a cesarean should be applauded for their success in coping with their recovery and a tiny baby as well. It is natural to be depressed following any major operation, especially a cesarean, when the body is undergoing hormonal changes as well as healing. Some women are temporarily depressed following natural childbirth, too, because of hormonal changes.

It is also understandable not to feel affection for the baby when you are tired and probably have some discomfort. Talk things over with your doctor. You could try talking to other new mothers, who will understand and sympathize with your feelings.

If my sister has had one cesarean birth, will she have to have another with her next baby?

It depends why the operation was performed. For example, if she has a normal-size pelvis, and the operation was performed because the baby was distressed and there was no progress in labor, it is still possible for another pregnancy to result in a vaginal delivery.

My two children were born by cesarean section, and I would like a third child. Is there a limit to how many cesareans I can have before it becomes risky?

There is no limit. Each case is assessed by the obstetrician. With a third pregnancy, it is possible that he or she may advise early admission and early delivery to prevent strain.

A cesarean is a safe, speedy surgical operation that is performed when a natural delivery is not possible or desired. Either a general anesthetic is given or epidural anesthesia is used, with the mother remaining awake.

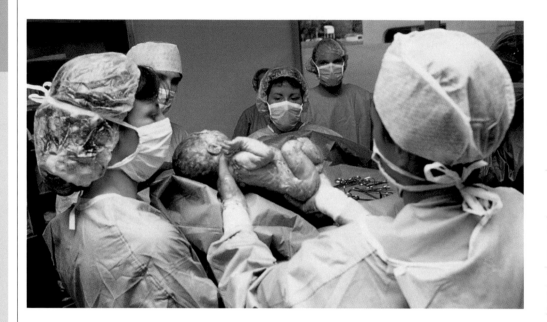

▲ *Approximately 25 to 30 percent of births in the United States are by cesarean section.*

A cesarean birth means that the baby is born through a surgical incision made in the mother's abdominal wall and uterus (womb). It may be performed either as an emergency, when the life and health of the mother or baby are at stake, or be planned in advance because the doctors know that natural birth is impossible or unsafe in the particular circumstances.

A planned cesarean

Although the timing depends on the reason for the operation, most women who are having a planned cesarean section enter the hospital when they are 38 weeks pregnant or before. Tests will make sure the baby is mature enough to be delivered without being harmed. The night before surgery, the mother will be examined, the pubic area shaved, and an enema given to clear her intestine. Blood samples will be taken in advance for grouping and cross-matching in case a blood transfusion is needed (see Blood Transfusion). If a general anesthetic is to be used, the mother will not eat or drink after midnight the night before surgery. Many hospitals do a cesarean section under epidural anesthesia, which is injected into the epidural space just behind the spinal cord to numb the area below. With an epidural, the mother can hold her baby immediately after birth, and the father may be allowed to watch the birth. If a woman knows she needs to have a cesarean section, she should ask for an epidural if she wants to be aware of what is happening.

Emergency cesareans

Although "emergency cesarean" sounds like a life-or-death situation, it rarely is. Once in the operating room, medical experts frequently perform the operation safely and deliver the baby in just five to seven minutes. Signs of possible problems with the baby are detected by external monitoring of the heart using a process called computerized ultrasound fetal cardiotocography (CTG). This simply involves placing a small, smooth detector (transducer) over the womb, or sometimes in the vagina. The results seen on the monitor provide a detailed account of the state of the activity of the fetal heart and an early indication of fetal distress. If a problem is detected, preparations for the operation are hasty. An intravenous infusion (drip) will be set up. Fluids are essential for the prevention of shock, and extra blood may be required through a blood transfusion. The abdomen and pubic area are quickly prepared by shaving before the anesthetic is given. With a general anesthetic, the mother-to-be will be unconscious (see Anesthetics). The bladder will be emptied with a catheter before surgery. The nurse-midwife checks the fetal heart on the monitor at regular intervals before the surgery begins. The father may not be permitted in the operating room, but he is usually allowed to sit nearby.

The operation

Nowadays most obstetricians—doctors who specialize in pregnancy and birth—make the incision in the lower part of the abdomen on the bikini line to minimize long-term weakening of the womb. An incidental advantage is a much less conspicuous scar. Retractors are inserted to hold back the layers of tissue. The lower segment of the womb is exposed, and the internal incision is widened. The doctor puts his or her hand into the womb to lift out the baby's head. (Forceps may be used to deliver the head.) The assistant presses the top of the womb to push the baby out. The placenta is delivered, and the mother is given a drug to contract the womb. The abdomen is then stitched. Meanwhile the baby is given immediately to the pediatrician, who is always present to check the newborn. The suddenness of the birth can cause the baby some shock, and it can take a few minutes for him or her to respond normally. It may take a while for the breathing to become regular and for the heart rate to steady. This situation is normal and need not cause concern. The baby can be lethargic because of the anesthetic given to the mother and may need drugs to counteract the effects. Most babies are put into an incubator to warm up and to be observed while the mother comes around from the anesthetic. If all is well, mother and baby can go back to the ward and both parents may hold and cuddle the baby.

Care of the mother

With a general anesthetic, it may be several hours before the mother's fatigue and nausea wear off. Some women even forget having seen their babies when they were first shown them by the doctor. The abdomen is very tender for several days, and it is difficult for the woman to move at first. An IV line may have been put in place after the operation, and it will stay in, perhaps for several days, until the gut is working properly. It may also take the mother time to urinate easily. Pain relief will be available and may be needed at first. The mother can breast-feed her baby before she takes pain-relief injections, so that there is a minimal drug effect on the baby. Tiredness does ease, but feeding can be exhausting to start with. If a mother does not want her baby to have formula milk, she can request breast milk from the milk bank if it is available. Or she can express her own milk.

HOW A CESAREAN DELIVERY IS PERFORMED

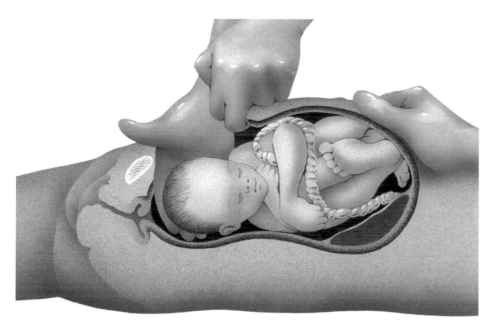

Reasons for an emergency cesarean
BEFORE LABOR, AS A RESULT OF UNEXPECTED BLEEDING DUE TO:
Separation of placenta from uterine (womb) wall.
Placenta previa—this is when the placenta has grown across the neck of the womb (cervix). The cervix opens up before labor and the placenta starts to detach, with bleeding.
THE BABY IS SUFFERING FROM:
Fetal distress—this shows up on the monitor. The baby's heartbeat may slow, or quicken, and become irregular.
Lack of oxygen due to prolapse of the umbilical cord. The cord comes out through the vagina ahead of the baby, and the change in temperature makes the blood vessels in the cord contract, cutting off the blood supply to the baby.
Pressure on the cord, which stops oxygen from being carried to the baby.
DURING LABOR, OWING TO THE MOTHER'S EXHAUSTION BECAUSE OF:
Poor or no progress in labor.
High blood pressure—the mother may be prone to this condition anyway, or it may have been caused by health difficulties during pregnancy.
Failed induction of labor. If labor is started artificially by breaking the water and giving a drug that stimulates contractions, and this attempt fails, the operation is necessary to avoid harm to mother and baby.
ALSO:
Mother has active genital herpes, and passage of baby through the birth canal would expose him or her to a potentially fatal infection.

◄ *An abdominal incision is made, and the doctor puts his or her hand into the womb and lifts out the baby's head while an assistant presses the top of the womb to help the baby out.*

Why a planned cesarean may be necessary

The outlet of the pelvis is smaller than the baby's head.
Abnormalities of the pelvis would prevent natural birth.
There is a disease that would endanger the mother's life if she gave birth naturally, such as a heart or lung disease.
There has been a previous cesarean birth.
Breech presentation—the baby is positioned feet or bottom first. Breech presentation can prolong labor and put strain on a scar from a previous cesarean section.

Getting up and walking on the second day is advised because of the risk of blood clots in the legs. The mother will be encouraged to get up for a few minutes even on the first day. She should not be surprised if she feels exhausted. The tube in the bladder and the IV line will be removed if all is well. Sometimes there is a small drainage tube in the wound, but this is usually taken out after 48 hours. Most hospitals have visiting physiotherapists who may suggest chest exercises to prevent infection and static blood flow due to inactivity. The mother may still want pain relief, but this need will soon pass.

The mother will now have more energy. She may have a bath with help. If there is a problem going to the bathroom, a suppository—a pill inserted in the rectum—may be given. This helps relieve the distention and discomfort often felt after abdominal surgery. The clips or sutures are usually taken out on the sixth day, but this will be done on an outpatient basis after discharge at four days.

Long-term effects

A woman may find that it is several months before she feels really well, and this is quite natural. She may find the wound from the operation tender and sore for some weeks, and bending and lifting may be difficult. Planning for help at home is essential for at least a few weeks. The baby's father may be able to do more around the home than usual during this time, or a relative might come to stay.

Postnatal exercises may be too uncomfortable to do at first, but they can be done later. Sometimes it takes time to urinate for a few weeks, owing to a loss of bladder tone, which will return. Sexual intercourse can be uncomfortable while the wound is sore, but discomfort can also be due to tenderness of the internal pelvic organs, which have been handled during surgery. If discomfort is prolonged, advice should be sought from the doctor or the hospital.

Emotional problems

Many women feel they have failed by not having a natural birth. But having a cesarean section and coping with a new baby are far from failing. Usually the excitement of the baby overrides the fact that there was a major operation. Partners and relatives need to remember that the mother needs special help, care, and attention.

If there were complications and the mother was separated from the baby after the operation, delayed early contact may mean that she finds it harder to bond with the baby. This is especially so if she

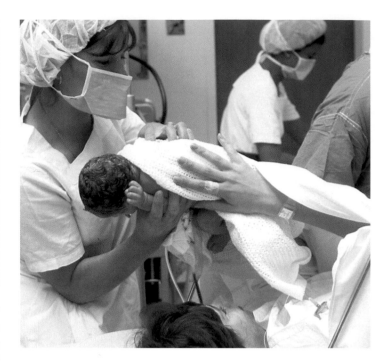

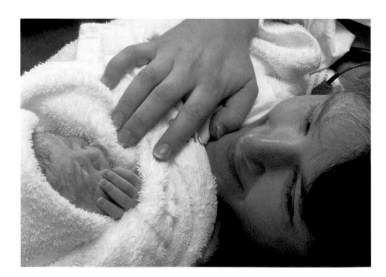

▲▼ *A woman can have an epidural anesthetic for a cesarean and be conscious during the birth. She is handed the baby immediately afterward (above) and is able to hold and cuddle the infant (below) even while the doctor stitches her incision.*

feels sore and in temporary pain and discomfort. It is natural not to feel immediately close to the baby after a cesarean birth, and temporary depression is perfectly normal too. Only when these feelings continue for a long time will expert help be needed.

Faint scarring

The operation scar is permanent, but it fades slightly. If the incision was made at the bikini line, it will not be noticeable. If necessary, the scar can be removed by plastic surgery, but a woman should not do this if she wants more children, in case a future delivery should result in another cesarean.

See also: **Birth; Breech birth; Enema; Intravenous infusion; Pregnancy; Uterus; Vagina**

Chat Room

My teenage daughter spends a lot of time in chat rooms. I have become worried by reports of child abuse by pedophiles who make a relationship with youngsters online and then persuade them to meet. What can I do to make sure the chat rooms she uses are suitable?

Before your daughter uses a chat room, consider the following:
• Is the chat room supervised? Who are the supervisors?
• Does the chat room have clear terms and conditions of use?
• Does the chat room have a clear topic timetable?
• Does the chat room have advertising or external links?
• Are there enough opportunities for young people to interact and shape the chat?
• Can anyone join or is there access control and password verification?
• Does the chat room discuss safety issues (such as not giving out personal information and not meeting a new friend offline without a trusted adult present)?

Is there specific web etiquette for chat rooms? What does it entail?

Yes, there are a number of rules for using a chat room. First, if it caters to a specific subject, stay on that subject. If you are in a history chat room, for example, do not start talking about sports. Second, do not get involved in arguments —if a conversation gets abusive or out of hand, leave the area. However, always announce when you are leaving a chat room—it is not polite to just disappear. Also, do not give out your name and address or any revealing personal information such as clubs you belong to. Other rules include not "shouting" (typing using upper-case letters) and not pairing off with any one person in the chat room. If you wish to talk in depth to an individual, enter a private room or use Instant Messaging— a form of messaging software for chats between two people.

A "chat room" is an Internet site that allows people to exchange typed messages to create a dialogue. Chat rooms can focus on diverse topics on an educational, recreational, or social theme, and they are particularly popular among young people.

A chat room is a virtual room—a "room" on the Internet—where two or more people can meet to "chat" (through typed messages) and share ideas, often on a specified topic. In a chat room the messages a person types are shown instantly to every other member of the "room." Therefore, a person can have a typed conversation with others in real time—something that is not possible with E-mail or bulletin boards.

When used correctly, chat rooms can be both informative and supportive. People who may have suffered a death in the family, for example, are able to log on to any one of a number of chat rooms whose members have been through a similar experience. They can use the chat room to talk about how they feel, and to give support to and receive support from other members. Similarly, people who have an interest in gardening can log onto a chat room for gardeners where they can ask questions of other members, exchange tips and advice, and so on. There are numerous chat rooms on the Internet that cover just about any topic, from modern art to travel, from health concerns to child-rearing and education.

Positive benefits

Chat rooms can also be a lot of fun. People logging onto a chat room do not always have a special topic they wish to discuss. This is particularly true of children and teenagers, who often log onto the Internet so that they can chat with their friends or other young people they have met online.

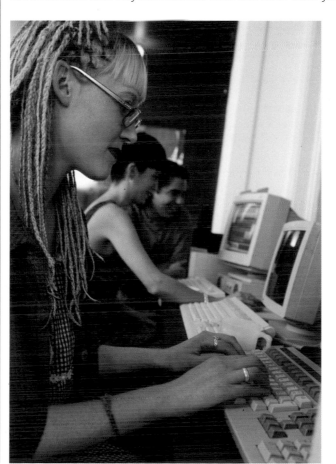

Subjects are much as they would be with any teenage discussion —music, television, films, sport, boyfriends and girlfriends, and so on. A chat room can be very good for young people in that it allows them to talk to and develop relationships with people who live all over the world. It also provides a medium through which children can communicate with people of their own age who have similar interests and concerns, and where they are able to talk in real time with family, friends, and teachers. In addition, chat rooms provide good practice in writing and expression.

◄ *Students are often drawn to chat rooms because the rooms provide good educational opportunities, as well as a social outlet where students can communicate via their computers with many people all over the world.*

Common symbols and abbreviations used in chat rooms								
>:-<	Angry		:-[	Pouting		BRB	Be right back
(::()::)	Bandaid; offering help		:(	Sad		FAQ	Frequently asked questions
:*)	Clowning		:O	Shocked		ICN	I see now
:'	Crying		:-V	Shouting		IOW	In other words
:-6	Exhausted; wipeout		:-)	Smiling; agreeing		J/K	Just kidding
}{	Face-to-face		:-,	Smirk		JMO	Just my opinion
:-(	Frowning; boo hoo		^	Thumbs up		L8R	Later
:^D	"Great! I like it."		:-\	Undecided		LOL	Laughing out loud
:-|	Grim		:@	What?		LTNS	Long time no see
[ ]	Hugs		;-)	Winking; just kidding		MSG	Message
: *	Kisses		AFK	Away from keyboard		TTYL	Talk to you later
:-D	Laughing		BAK	Back at keyboard		P2P	Person to person
:-X	My lips are sealed		BBL	Be back later		WB	Welcome back

Some major chat rooms can be found on search engines and Internet service providers such as Yahoo, MSN, and AOL. In some cases whole sites are devoted to chat, such as TalkCity.com and ChatWeb.net. People wishing to visit a chat room must first register and download a small chat application (this should take no more than a minute or so). They can then start receiving and sending messages to or from the group of people whose names appear on their screen.

Potential dangers

Despite the benefits, parents, teachers, politicians, and law enforcement agencies are increasingly anxious about the potential risks to young people who use chat rooms. It is important for parents to ensure that their children use chat rooms which are specifically set up for young people and which are monitored by trained adults (as they are at Teen.com, for example). These supervisors oversee all conversations and deal with bad language, racism, and abuse. In chat rooms other than these, children may be exposed to offensive language and adult conversation. They might also come across advertising or other links that might draw them away from the group, perhaps to sites that contain pornography or other unsuitable material. Parents must also consider the subjects that their children are discussing online. Adult-monitored chat rooms will deter youngsters from broaching topics such as sex and drugs, for example.

However, the main danger is that chat rooms—because of their interactive nature—are the most likely online activity through which children might meet people who wish to harm them. Pedophiles are known to log onto chat rooms used by young people, concealing their true identity and often pretending to be another teenager so as to gain the trust of a child. Eventually they may attempt to lure the child into meeting them offline. Research has shown that one child in every five using the Internet has been the victim of a sexual approach. Most of those approaches were initiated in chat rooms.

Reducing the risks

Parents need to carry out a number of safety measures to reduce the risks to which their child is exposed when he or she is chatting online. First, they should accompany the child in chat rooms until he or she learns the safety rules. Second, parents should teach their child never to give out personal information, such as his or her name, address, phone number, E-mail address, town, school, or any other information by which the child might be identified. Parents need to explain that people are not always who they say they are. Anyone can pretend to be a child or a teenager. Most important, children must never arrange to meet anyone in person without a parent or another trusted adult present. Parents may wish to limit their child to specific chat rooms, or may consider forbidding chat rooms altogether.

Some of the larger Internet sites, such as Yahoo, are considering appointing specially trained inspectors to monitor chat rooms and other websites for their use by suspected pedophiles. The British government has proposed that chat-room operators provide children with "panic buttons"—keys the children could press on their keyboards if they suspected they were being approached by a pedophile—which would then alert service providers to the potential danger. Some safeguards are already in place, however. If a chat-room user is wary of another chat-room member, he or she can click on the name of that member, then click on the Ignore User icon. Any messages sent by that member will then be blocked.

Parents should be aware that too much time spent online, even when that time is closely monitored, can limit a child's development. It may begin to take the place of schoolwork, friends, sports, and other activities. Therefore, parents might wish to consider putting a time limit on their child's Internet use each day.

> **See also: Adolescence; Drug abuse; Grief; Group therapy; Sex; Sexual abuse**

Chelation therapy

Chelation is a treatment that attempts to rid the body of heavy metals which have accumulated there and which threaten the patient's health. It is used to treat lead or mercury poisoning and, more recently, calcified blocked arteries.

Chelation therapy is based on the principle that some substances are able to bind to others. Chelating agents such as the synthetically produced drugs amino acid ethylenediaminetetra-acetate (EDTA), sodium dimercapto-propane sulfonate (DMPS), and meso-2,3-dimercapto-succinic acid (DMSA) have this ability. When the chelating agent meets harmful, toxic metals in the body, such as lead, mercury, cadmium, and aluminum, it engulfs them then excretes them in body wastes.

How chelation works

In the case of heavy-metal poisoning, the chelating agent attacks positively charged metal ions by surrounding them and making them inactive before removing them from the body. It is not known exactly how chelation works on patients with atherosclerosis (calcified blocked arteries), but two theories exist (see Arteries and Artery Disease).

The first involves the parathyroid glands, which control calcium levels in the bloodstream (see Parathyroid Glands). When the chelating agent appears in the bloodstream, blood calcium levels are lowered, causing the parathyroid hormone to be released in large quantities. The hormone may help dissolve the plaque in the arteries, but this has not yet been proved.

The second theory concerns free radicals, which are molecules that arise in the body both naturally and unnaturally. Because they have unpaired electrons, they are highly charged and unstable and can cause much damage. Free radicals are thought to increase in the presence of metallic elements and irritate the lining of the blood vessels. Chelating agents remove the metallic irritants and allow the damaged walls to heal. The walls of the arteries become softer and more pliable, and there is increased blood flow.

Another reason chelation may improve cardiac symptoms is that it removes heavy metals such as lead and cadmium, which can contribute to hypertension and lead to heart disease.

Development of chelation techniques

From the mid-1950s until 2001, chelation was mainly administered intravenously (IV), orally, or intramuscularly (IM); most treatment was intravenous, with EDTA as the chelating agent. Now the therapy is available in the form of EDTA suppositories. This means that the patient can take the treatment anywhere, without spending several hours at a doctor's office or a hospital, as in the IV method.

The history of EDTA

EDTA was first used as an industrial cleaning agent in Germany in the 1930s to clean pipes in textile mills. Then in Detroit, Michigan, in the 1950s it was found to be effective in cleansing the bodies of workers in the auto trade who were contaminated with lead. Dr. Norman Clarke, who carried out the procedure, noticed that patients who also had coronary heart disease experienced improvement of their cardiac symptoms after lead was removed from their bodies. However, using chelation to treat atherosclerosis still creates controversy.

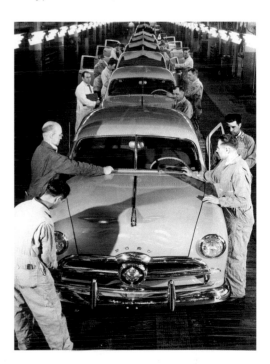

▲ *Chelation was used in the 1950s to cure auto industry workers of lead poisoning.*

CHELATION THERAPY

Typical EDTA intravenous procedure

First an hour-long ultrasonic investigation, called a bidirectional Doppler examination, is made on the main arterial sites leading to the patient's brain and legs (see Ultrasound). The test reveals any deposits or obstructions in the arteries that could impair blood flow or break away and cause strokes. It also shows any hardening inside the brain's capillaries that could cause memory loss. A blood test is then taken to determine the individual's blood sugar and cholesterol levels and the state of the liver and kidneys. A urine test is also conducted to establish the kidneys' condition. Finally, an electrocardiograph (ECG) is taken to determine the state of the heart.

Once these tests have been completed, the chelation practitioner can determine the length of the patient's chelation treatment on the basis of the results. An average of 20 to 30 IV infusions of EDTA will be needed, usually given once a week, and each lasting about three and a half hours. In some cases the patient may require as many as 100 treatments. Because chelation therapy may deplete the body of vital minerals, such as zinc, magnesium, calcium, manganese, and selenium, along with toxic metals, the patient will be advised to take vitamin and mineral supplements during treatment. He or she will also be told to eat a nutritious diet that is low in fat and highly refined and processed food, to avoid tobacco, and to exercise regularly.

Intramuscular treatment

Intramuscular (IM) chelation treatment is now the least common form. It involves a series of painful injections of dimercaprol (BAL) taken along with an intravenous treatment of EDTA.

DMSA oral chelation

DMSA is rich in sulfur—a strong magnet for toxic metals—and is taken orally. It is considered to be the most effective chelation treatment for mercury poisoning. However, DMSA must be taken with at least 1½ quarts (1.5 l) of water per day to avoid kidney damage, and for no more than three days per week for three weeks, with a week off to protect the liver.

DMPS chelation

DMPS, which can be taken either orally or intravenously, is considered the least safe and least effective form of chelation. It is three times more toxic than DMSA and has more unpleasant side effects than any other chelation treatment. Not until 1999 did the FDA officially allow this type of treatment. However, it is considered to be the most effective chelation method for eliminating mercury from the kidneys.

EDTA suppositories

EDTA suppositories are patented and marketed under the name Detoxamin. They cost about 70 percent less than IV chelation treatments and, unlike DMSA and DMPS, are available without a prescription. Each suppository takes only 30 seconds to administer once a day before bedtime. Advocates of EDTA suppositories claim that they are more effective than IV chelation because they bypass the liver and go directly to the body's organs, and more effective than oral chelation because the rectum is less acidic than the stomach and enzymatic degradation does not occur (see Suppositories). They are also thought to be better for mercury detoxification because they reach the large intestine—where most of the body's mercury resides—more quickly than other chelation methods.

Potential dangers

Possible side effects from IV chelation include decreased appetite and lethargy. Side effects of DMSA can include nausea and vomiting, diarrhea or constipation, rashes, itches, rhinitis, mucositis, coughing, and fever. DMPS has the largest number of side effects, including pancreatis (inflammation of the pancreas), nausea, diarrhea, stomach pain, headaches, muscle pain or weakness, rashes, decreased urination, cardiac arrhythmias (heart beating too fast or too slowly), and allergic reactions. All types of chelation therapy can result in a weakened immune system if supplements are not taken to counteract this effect (see Immune System).

Another theoretical danger causing concern among some doctors is that since chelation draws toxic metals out of the cells and bones and into the bloodstream before excreting them, there is a chance that the chelating agent may not be able to retain its bond on all the metals it has gathered up and may drop them suddenly in a lump within the bloodstream, where they can poison the immune and nervous system, as well as vital organs (see Nervous System). The body has a natural tendency to closet metals away in areas where they will do less harm, and chelation may disturb this form of natural protection if the chelating agent is not entirely effective in its bonding process.

Chelation versus surgery for atherosclerosis

Critics of chelation argue that it is not tried and tested for atherosclerosis. In its defense, practitioners have commented that, given the very nature of conventional medical procedures, its effectiveness cannot be tested by a controlled trial. However, its success rate in patients suffering from atherosclerosis is claimed to be close to 82 percent. More than 400,000 patients have received chelation therapy over 6 million times, and no sustained serious side effects from the treatment have been reported. A minority of physicians believe that chelation therapy is an acceptable method of treatment for atherosclerosis and that, when administered according to an accepted standard of practice, it is safer than surgical bypass and angioplasty procedures, which carry a much greater risk of fatality, usually from strokes and heart attacks. An average of 4 percent of people who undergo bypass surgery die during the operation. Another 4 to 5 percent die in the first year—this figure increases to 15 percent in people over 65—and 5 percent suffer from long-lasting or permanent cerebral damage. For every 1,000 people who undergo balloon angioplasty operations, five die and 8 percent suffer from permanent renal failure. Therefore some doctors feel that balloon angioplasty and bypass surgery, which are among the most common procedures in the United States, are unjustified in many cases. The surgery does not change the biochemistry that causes the degeneration of the arteries, and unless it is backed up by changes in lifestyle and nutrition, it does not seem to have a lasting effect.

Chelation treatment also has the advantage that it is relatively inexpensive compared with balloon angioplasty and bypass surgery. The treatment costs less than 10 percent of what surgery costs.

See also: **Blood; Cholesterol; Electrocardiogram; Heart attack; Heart disease; Intravenous infusion; Kidneys and kidney diseases; Lead poisoning; Lethargy; Liver and liver diseases; Pancreas and disorders; Stroke**

Chest

Questions and Answers

I am an avid gardener, but I get pains in my chest after I have been digging. Could this mean that I have strained my heart?

Probably not, because most chest pains are the result of muscle strains in the chest wall. The chest provides the platform from which our arms and shoulders do all their muscular work, so it is not surprising that we sometimes strain or pull the chest muscles. The clue is usually the fact that a specific movement or set of movements will bring on the pain. To put your mind at rest, see your doctor.

I broke my ribs playing basketball, but I was not bandaged or given any treatment. Why was this?

Although broken or cracked ribs can be uncomfortable or painful, the main danger is that the chest movement will be reduced, producing less airflow into and out of the underlying lung. This can cause pneumonia, so it is unusual to bandage broken ribs.

My doctor says I am pigeon-chested. What is this? And am I more likely to get chest infections?

Minor deformities of the chest wall are often referred to as a pigeon chest. The most common form is a hollowing of the center of the chest at the front, but this does not mean that you are more liable to chest infection.

Can people still die of pneumonia as they did in the old days?

Unfortunately, yes. Pneumonia used to be a common cause of death not so many years ago, even in healthy young people, but generally this is no longer the case. However, in people who are seriously ill for some other reason, or are elderly, pneumonia is often the final illness that kills them.

The bony, muscular structure of the chest forms a protective framework around two of the body's most important organs, the lungs and the heart. It is essential to know when a cough or chest pain needs medical attention.

The chest is a bony cage that contains two of the most important organs in the body: the lungs and the heart. The basic function of these organs is to transfer oxygen from the air to the tissues, where it is essential for the continuation of life (see Heart; Lung and Lung Diseases).

The bell-shaped rib cage is located just under the skin of the chest. It encloses the lungs and heart on all but their lowest surface. It is attached to the spine at the back, and its base is sealed off by the diaphragm, the thick muscular sheet separating the chest from the abdomen. In between the ribs are further muscular sheets called the intercostal ("between the ribs") muscles. The chest wall thus consists of a bell-shaped muscular bag with the ribs as struts. By expanding and contracting it sucks air in and out through the windpipe, or trachea, which emerges into the neck.

A membrane called the pleura lines the whole of the inside of the chest, and similar membranes cover the lungs and the heart. When the pleura becomes inflamed, this leads to pleurisy.

The two lungs fill the bulk of the chest and are connected by their tubes, the main bronchi, to the trachea. Smaller tubes, or bronchioles, split off from each main bronchus like branches of a tree, carrying air to the air sacs (alveoli). Here oxygen is extracted from the air and passed into the blood, while carbon dioxide—the body's waste product—moves in the opposite direction.

The heart lies at the front of the chest between the two lungs, inside its own membranous bag. It receives blood from the body through the pumping chambers on its right side (the right atrium

ORGANS OF THE CHEST

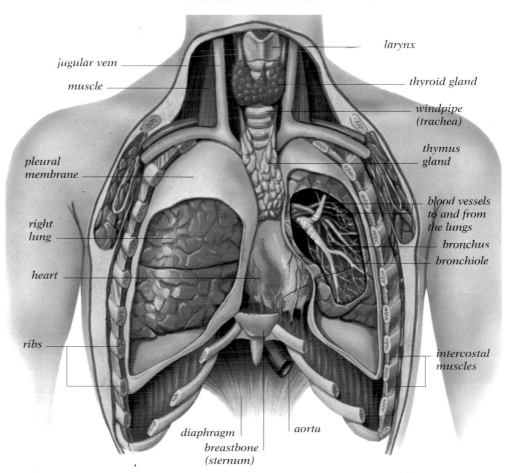

- larynx
- jugular vein
- muscle
- thyroid gland
- windpipe (trachea)
- thymus gland
- pleural membrane
- blood vessels to and from the lungs
- right lung
- bronchus
- bronchiole
- heart
- ribs
- intercostal muscles
- diaphragm
- aorta
- breastbone (sternum)

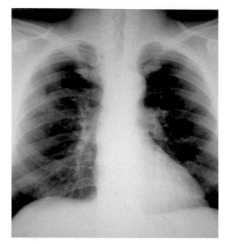

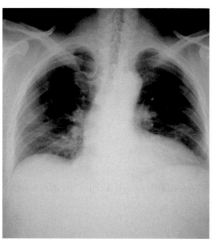

▲ *These X rays show how the muscular walls of the chest expand when air is inhaled (top) and contract when it is exhaled (above).*

Pain in the chest: When to see your doctor

TYPE OF PAIN	OTHER SIGNS	CAUSES
Central pain, pressing and dull in character.	Breathlessness, nausea, or sweating, lasting more than 20 minutes.	Angina (heart disease). Heart attack. Pericarditis (inflammation of the membrane lining the heart). Indigestion.
Central, gripping pain spreading to the neck, shoulders, or arms.	Brought on by exercise or emotional excitement.	Angina. Pericarditis.
Anywhere, worse on inspiration (breathing in) or on coughing.	May be associated with a cough or an attack of bronchitis.	Pleurisy. Pericarditis.
Central, burning. Worse after food or on bending forward; may be worse at night.	Foods may bring it on, and it may be relieved by milk or indigestion tablets.	Esophagitis (inflammation of the gullet, a form of indigestion).

When a cough needs medical attention

TYPE OF COUGH	CAUSE
Green or yellow sputum coughed up.	Bronchitis (inflammation of the lining of the bronchial tubes in the lungs) or pneumonia (inflammation of the lung).
Cough or wheezing.	This may be true asthma or wheezy bronchitis.
Coughing up blood or bloody streaks in sputum.	There are many causes of this, but the most serious are tuberculosis or lung cancer.

and ventricle) and pumps the blood into the lungs. Blood full of oxygen returns from the lungs to the left atrium and ventricle, from where it is pumped out into the main artery of the body—the aorta.

The chest also contains the gullet, or esophagus, which carries food from the mouth to the stomach. At the top of the chest in front of the windpipe is the thymus gland. It is important in the maturation of immune system cells but virtually disappears before adulthood.

Chest problems

Chest complaints have three main symptoms: pain, coughing, and breathlessness (see Coughing). Pain in the chest may arise from the chest wall, as a result of pleurisy and various other conditions, or it may arise from the heart. The esophagus may also be the source of pain, since the acid contents of the stomach may wash back upward, causing inflammation. In cases of pleurisy, the two layers of pleura lining the inside of the chest and outside of the lungs become inflamed and cause pain when they rub together. The pain of pleurisy is worse on deep breathing or coughing (see Pleurisy).

Since the lungs do not give direct pain signals, coughing is an important symptom of damage to the lung. Doctors call a cough "productive" when it produces phlegm or sputum. This may indicate infection, particularly if the sputum is green or yellow rather than white. Most coughs, however, do not produce sputum and are simply a result of inflammation of the upper airways rather than a sign of lung disease. Such coughs usually follow a cold.

Breathlessness may be a result of disease of either the lungs or the chest. Asthma is a common cause, particularly in younger people and children, and is accompanied by wheezing. Heart problems lead to breathlessness because the reduced blood circulation cannot carry the amount of oxygen required by the body; the lungs move stiffly because they are somewhat distended with blood. This situation is referred to as heart failure and is common in the elderly. In its most serious form, known as pulmonary edema, it can be life-threatening.

Urgent medical advice is needed if a person experiences a new, severe pain in the chest, shoulders, or arms, especially if there is breathlessness, nausea, and sweating, or if breathing or coughing makes the pain worse. Prompt advice is also needed if a cough produces phlegm or is accompanied by wheezing, if blood is coughed up, if there are bloody streaks in the sputum, or if there is extreme breathlessness with a bubbling cough.

See also: **Asthma; Phlegm**

Chicken pox

Children catch chicken pox so easily that it is almost a natural hazard of childhood. Fortunately, the illness does not last long and rarely has serious complications, so effective home nursing is a simple matter.

Questions and Answers

What is the best way to prevent scars forming from chicken pox? Both my older children scratched their spots, and it would be a shame if my daughter were to scar her face when she gets it.

Scarring occurs if the spots become infected or if the scabs are pulled off, taking fresh tissue with them and widening the area of damage. Preventing itching with calamine lotion or an antihistamine drug is helpful, but it does take willpower not to scratch. All you can do is explain what will happen if she picks the spots, and encourage her to resist the temptation.

Could my baby daughter get chicken pox, and if so, is it more serious than in an older child?

Babies seem to have some natural immunity to chicken pox, and few cases have ever been recorded. A baby could be seriously, but probably not fatally, ill with chicken pox—but any child under the age of two who develops a rash should be seen by a doctor.

My brother appears to have chicken pox for the second time. Is this possible?

It is unlikely. In general, chicken pox is a one-time-only infection. The first "attack" might have been scabies (severe itching and spots caused by a mite) or several gnat bites occurring together.

My daughter recently spent the day with a child who now has chicken pox. How soon will she come down with it?

Your daughter may show the first symptoms—headache and a vague illness—within 10 days, or it could take up to three weeks to develop. But she may not develop chicken pox at all—there is no certainty that she was infected.

Chicken pox—the medical name is varicella—is a highly infectious illness, easily recognized by the rash that it causes (see Rashes). It is generally considered a childhood illness. Babies are born with a natural ability (passed on by their mothers) to resist chicken pox, but this wears off by the time children are three or four years of age, leaving them vulnerable to infection.

The virus (germ) that causes chicken pox also causes shingles (which has similar symptoms, including a rash) in adults, so an adult with shingles can pass chicken pox on to a child. The virus is so infectious that many outbreaks of chicken pox occur, mainly in children between the ages of two and six. Outbreaks are strongest in the autumn and winter and appear to occur in three- or four-year cycles as the number of children who have never had the disease builds up.

Although slightly similar in appearance to smallpox, chicken pox has nothing else in common with the disease. Smallpox is much more serious, with a 40 percent death rate, and is caused by a completely different virus. It was eradicated more than 20 years ago (see Smallpox).

How it is caught

Although the chicken pox virus is present and alive in the spots that form, it is transferred between people chiefly by droplet infection. Someone who already has the virus spreads clusters of it in the tiny droplets of water that are exhaled with every breath. When a child breathes in an infected droplet, the virus starts to multiply, and another case of chicken pox begins. The source is almost always another child. The illness is usually passed on before the skin spots appear, so the affected child is not suspected as a source—hence the rapid spread.

Symptoms

Once the virus enters the body, it needs an incubation, or breeding, period of between 10 days and three weeks to spread. The first a child will know of his or her illness will be a 24-hour period when there will be symptoms of a vague headache, a sick feeling, occasional slight fever, and sometimes a blotchy, red rash that fades. A parent may note that the child is pale. Within 24 hours the first spots appear, and the nature and position of these spots allow a diagnosis to be made. In very mild cases it can be difficult to distinguish chicken pox from gnat bites, but in a full-blown case, with hundreds of spots, the diagnosis is simple.

Spots first appear in the mouth and throat, where they quickly burst, causing pain and soreness. They then appear on the trunk and face, only occasionally affecting the limbs. Each spot starts as a pink pimple, and within five or six hours becomes raised to form a tiny blister, or vesicle, containing clear fluid that is full of the virus. These teardrop spots gradually become milky in color, forming a crust and finally a scab. The time from the appearance of the teardrop to the formation of the crust is about 24 hours. During this period the child may be agitated and uncomfortable, and run a temperature of 100° or 101°F (38°C).

Some children have only a few spots, while others may have several hundred. As soon as crusts form, the spots begin to itch, and this stage may last until the scabs drop off, leaving

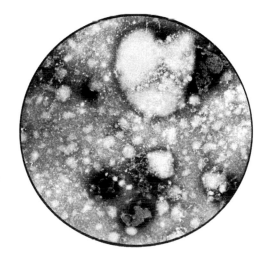

▲ *The chicken pox virus, enlarged about 8,000 times, is mainly transmitted through droplets of water in the breath.*

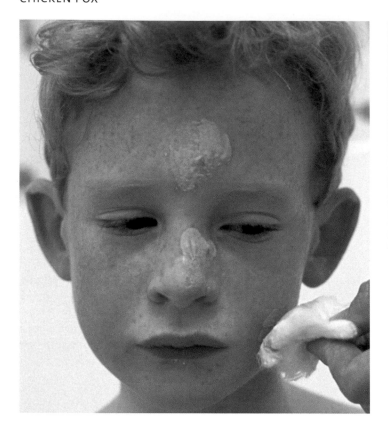

▲ *Chicken pox spots begin to itch as soon as the crusts form, and calamine lotion is a soothing, cooling treatment.*

Home care of a child

Reassure the child, allow him or her freedom, and do not insist on bed rest. Give mild painkillers for a sore throat or headache. The spots may look dramatic, but the child is rarely very sick.

Consult your doctor if the spots are very large, infected, or extremely painful (for instance, in the ear).

If the child is not hungry, cut down on food when temperature is high, but offer plenty of fluids.

Explain the need not to scratch, and suggest that the child might like to wear soft cotton gloves as a reminder.

Apply calamine lotion to reduce irritation, or ask the doctor for an antihistamine drug, which will have the same effect.

Make sure strict hygiene is observed—short nails, clean hands, and a daily bath at the scab stage.

Check with the school about isolation of the child. Usually a week is required from the appearance of the spots.

It can be reassuring for your child to ask another child with chicken pox to come to the house to play.

new skin after one or two weeks. Chicken pox spots come out in crops, which means that new ones appear every day for three or four days. When examining a child's skin, an adult will notice that the spots will be at different stages even in the same area.

In most cases the condition is mild, but in some cases the child is very sick and needs attentive home nursing.

Dangers

In children dangerous complications are rare, and most children with chicken pox feel well enough to play. Those who are taking steroid drugs or who are suffering from leukemia are the only ones likely to be seriously affected, and for them the condition can be fatal. In a small number of cases the virus can lead to a severe form of pneumonia.

Chicken pox can be dangerous in pregnant women, as it can affect the developing fetus, so a woman who has not had chicken pox should be vaccinated against it before becoming pregnant. In adults chicken pox pneumonia is fatal in more than 20 percent of cases.

Complications

The most common complications arise from infection of the spots, causing boils or other skin conditions. Similarly, spots near the eye may lead to infective conjunctivitis, commonly called pinkeye. In such cases treatment with antibiotics is needed.

Cases of arthritis and inflammation of the heart have followed chicken pox, but they are rare. The other danger arises when the virus attacks the nervous system and causes encephalitis (inflammation of the brain), as it may do on the fourth or tenth day after the rash appears. The patient becomes delirious, and intensive hospital treatment is needed. The chance of complete recovery is high.

Treatment

Children with a high temperature who feel unwell may prefer to stay in bed or lie downstairs to be with the family. Otherwise, there is no medical reason to enforce strict bed rest. Any pain from a sore throat or a headache is best relieved with a painkiller such as acetaminophen, or aspirin, in a child over 12. As there is no medical cure for the virus, the condition is left to take its natural course, and most children require no treatment at all.

Severe itching can be helped by applying calamine lotion, which has a cooling and anti-itching effect, or with an antihistamine drug. If any of the spots should become infected, they may take longer to heal, and antibiotics will be necessary.

Outlook

Most children who have had a mild case of chicken pox start losing their scabs after about 10 days and will be free of spots within about two weeks. If scabs have been scratched, the process takes a little longer. The scabs are not infectious and those that fall off do not leave a scar. Scabs that have been picked or have become infected are more likely to scar, so it is important to avoid scratching.

Chicken pox infection produces a lifelong immunity to the disease, but the virus remains in the body and can lead to shingles, which may develop later in a person's life (see Shingles).

A vaccine has now been developed for chicken pox, and this will probably become one of the standard set of childhood injections.

See also: **Blisters; Boils; Conjunctivitis; Encephalitis; Leukemia; Pneumonia; Steroids; Viruses**

Child abuse

Questions and Answers

I know my neighbor beats her son. I've seen terrible bruises on his face and arms. Whom should I contact?

A doctor or social worker will give practical help, and no one will know that it was you who contacted him or her. It would be better if you could offer some help yourself. Ask if you could look after the little boy; invite the mother in for coffee and get her to chat. Your friendship could make a lot of difference.

Will my child be taken away from me if it's discovered I've beaten her?

If you cooperate with the people who want to help you, and you manage to control your urges, then there is no danger that your child will be taken away. It is only as a last resort that children are placed in a foster home.

My husband has beaten our baby once or twice. Does he need help?

Yes, he does. To ignore his beating or to cover up for him can only be bad for the baby. Persuade him to see a doctor, who will refer him to someone who can help.

Sometimes I get really mad at my son. Will I end up beating him?

If you haven't done so before, the answer is probably no. Most abused babies are beaten in the first year of their life, and if you have managed to control your feelings so far, then you should be safe both now and in the future.

Can slapping develop into beating?

Physical violence to a child is never justified. If you find your child is driving you to distraction, get professional advice. Casual slapping can become a habit and can cross the line into child abuse.

Parents who abuse their children are likely to have suffered cruelty in childhood themselves, so they are emotionally damaged. How can they be helped—and what are the signs that a child is being abused?

"Child abuse" is a term used to describe the nonaccidental physical (including sexual) abuse of children by one or both parents or another adult, even though the children may be in all other respects well cared for and loved. Injuries can range from relatively minor to so serious that children die. Emotional abuse, in which children are taunted or told that they are not loved, or made to suffer mentally in other ways, often accompanies physical abuse, and the scars left from this can linger long after the body has healed.

Causes

Every parent has experienced helpless frustration in response to the nonstop crying of an infant who cannot be calmed. Most parents find that "something" stops them from hitting their child, but the lack of this internal psychological brake leads other parents to beat their children—not just once, but a number of times.

It is believed that as many as 20 percent of women experience difficulty in learning to become a mother. A small percentage of these go on to abuse their children, and the cause of this can be found far back in their own childhood.

Some child abusers of both sexes were beaten or sexually molested themselves as children, some are aggressive types with a pattern of physical violence in all their relationships, and others fall into neither group. Almost all were deprived of good parental care when they were children, so that they never learned to give and receive love and did not have a successful parent to model themselves on when the time came for them to raise their own children.

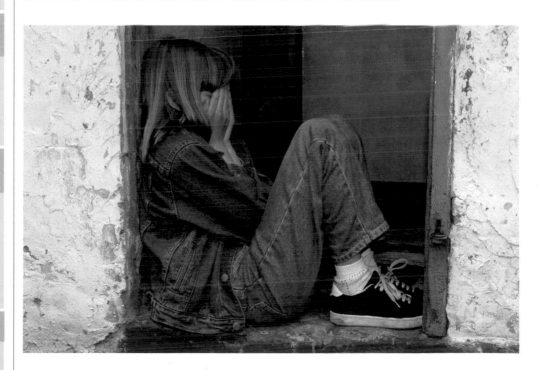

▲ *In 2000 the National Child Abuse and Neglect Data System recorded approximately 1,200 deaths related to child abuse and neglect. More than 3 million children were reported as victims of child abuse and neglect, and 879,000 cases of child maltreatment were identified; of these 63 percent were neglected, 19 percent were physically abused, 10 percent were sexually abused, and 8 percent were psychologically maltreated.*

Fewer than 10 percent of parents who abuse their children are severely psychologically ill, although half of the mothers who do so are classifiably neurotic and a third of fathers are said to have a gross personality defect. Many of them are depressed, passive, reclusive types who demand instant love from their children and fail to understand that for a long time babies are dependent and aware only of their own needs. Crying is interpreted as a sign that the baby does not love them, and the parents' feelings of anger and failure can trigger an attack. Other potential child abusers are obsessively clean and tidy, and a baby's natural soiling or a toddler's investigative messiness seem like deliberate naughtiness that must be punished (see Obsessive-Compulsive Disorder). A mother who has had to give up her career or put it on hold to have a child may also feel strong resentment and frustration.

Isolation is another contributing factor. A young mother whose own parents live far away, and who does not have friends nearby, may find that her desires and fears center on her baby, and she does not have the natural safety valve of talking with a sympathetic listener. If her marriage is also difficult or unhappy, then the baby will be even more at risk. Child abusers may be shocked and horrified at the damage they have caused while in a rage. Even though they may realize that they are placing unrealistic demands on their children, not even self-disgust will stop them from doing it again.

Social background

Research reveals that most child abuse is reported among the poor and deprived and that the level of intelligence of the abusing parent

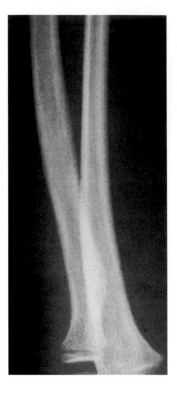

▶ *X ray showing child's forearm with a bent bone (right)—the result of a blow. A child's bones are soft and bend rather than break.*

is low. But statistics are compiled from cases that have come to the attention of the authorities—either from health visitors, social workers, hospitals, or the police—and experts are sure that the problem is more widespread.

Child abusers who are well-off are able to seek private treatment for their children. The more intelligent they are, and the higher their social class, the more easily they can deceive the authorities as to the true cause of their child's injuries. Doctors are also more disposed to believe the explanations of an articulate middle-class parent.

Some people also believe there is more chance that stepchildren or the children of single parents will be abused. But while these cases are represented in the statistics, most abuse occurs within normal family units. Another common supposition is that one child is singled out from a family group for beating. This is sometimes the case, but in most families where one child has been abused, other children suffer beatings too. One child may be be picked on at a particular time; and if the abusing parent is a good housekeeper, the clean, well-dressed appearance of the others makes them appear to be unharmed. Closer examination generally proves that, at different times, the others have also suffered unexplained injuries.

Anything is likely to trigger the violent rage of a harassed potential child abuser. However, some babies are more at risk: premature and underweight babies are in danger, because they need special care and patience and may be sickly and fretful, trying the patience of even the most well-meaning parent.

Emotional abuse

It is impossible to estimate the extent of emotional abuse when it occurs without physical injury. Parents who continually tell their children that they are clumsy, stupid, dishonest, unpleasant, or ugly do them great harm. The children begin to believe what is said of them, and it can affect their whole lives. If they are made to feel unloved, often they will unconsciously make themselves unlovable to other people, becoming antisocial. It is a vicious circle: a child's actions often make the parents feel that they are right, so they continue to hurt the child with words.

No physically abused child escapes an emotional battering either. Children who are hit repeatedly for real or imagined naughtiness live in fear. If physical contact means a blow as often as a hug, they may shrink from other people. Since it has been proved that children who are cuddled frequently tend to be mentally brighter, the implication for abused children is clear. Children who are beaten and then pampered by guilty parents will end up emotionally muddled and confused.

Preventing child abuse—A self-help guide

A baby has been crying all day and won't be comforted by her mother, or a toddler is aggravating his father. These are moments that any parent will recognize, when they feel themselves losing control and know they are in danger of lashing out. Punishment given in a blind rage can be dangerous—especially if the child is a baby.

Here are some suggestions that could help avert a crisis.

Work off aggression by working out at a gym. Spend time on the treadmill and lift some weights. The exercise may divert violent feelings.

Telephone someone and talk about any negative feelings.

Ask a neighbor or friend to watch the child for a while, and get out of the house. Walk and think until you feel calmer.

If getting out is not an option, go into a different room from the child. Go into the kitchen and make tea. Cry or shout. Giving angry feelings expression (without violence to the child) will make them go away faster.

When the feelings have passed, don't just hope that they will never occur again. Seek help from a doctor, nurse, or social worker. He or she will understand without being shocked and will offer practical aid and advice.

Symptoms

Identifying abused children is harder than it would seem. Most parents who abuse their children bring them for treatment voluntarily and are clearly distressed by the children's injuries. Usually, abused children are genuinely loved, the beating being performed in a rage by parents who have the emotional problems already mentioned. Some parents even have a partial memory blackout about the beating. They do not want to admit to themselves that they inflicted injuries on their own children, and they are often glib and convincing in explaining the "accident" that caused the injury. In other ways, the children may look well cared for, so the parent's explanation is often accepted. Alert doctors and teachers can spot the signs that indicate child abuse. Apart from the physical symptoms, a professional will notice if there is any delay in reporting an injury; even parents who bring their child in for treatment may wait a day or two before doing so. Another sign is the child's attitude: occasionally children may flinch from their parents, although some abused children are especially loving to their parents in an attempt to win their affection.

Actual injuries vary, but even when a reasonable excuse is given for the way in which the injuries happened, an examination can prove that the damage is inconsistent with, say, a fall downstairs or an accidental bang against a door frame. The most serious injuries are those to the face and head: fractured skulls or bruised and cut faces are often seen. Failure to thrive may be another sign. This is the term used for children who are underweight and not developing normally. Failure to thrive could indicate that they are neglected, but in the case of abused children, unhappiness could be the cause.

Children are abused in different ways, and the list makes unpleasant reading. Some are beaten on the head, punched, kicked, bitten, and thrown across a room or downstairs. Others are burned by cigarettes, thrown against fires, or even placed in ovens or boiling baths. Some parents confine themselves to shaking their children, believing that this does less harm—but young babies can suffer brain damage if shaken violently, even though their soft bones may sustain the shock of being thrown to the floor. Doctors look out for heavy bruising caused by tight gripping around the head or limbs while children are beaten or thrown. X rays can show old healed injuries or damage to internal organs (see Fractures).

Treatment

Physically curing abused children is the easiest part of the treatment, but it does not get to the root of the problem. According to some experts, severely abused children who are returned to their parents when the parents' problems have not been treated stand a 25 to 50 percent chance of being killed or permanently injured. Sixty percent will be abused again, and an even higher percentage will suffer minor attacks or emotional battering.

How can parents be treated to stop them from abusing their children? Certainly an increased knowledge of what to expect from their children at each stage of growth and development is a great help, along with practical aid with child-raising problems.

Doctors and social workers should recognize that sometimes the obvious nature of children's injuries is a cry for help from the parents, and it should be answered by offers of support rather than accusations and disgust. Above all, the best treatment enables the parents to relearn the art of loving and caring for their children, which is brought about by being loved and "mothered" themselves.

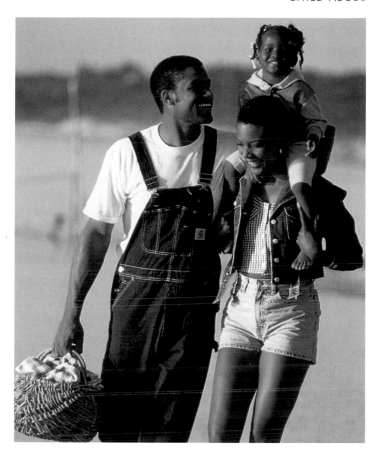

▲ *An abused child can be helped to recover physically and emotionally by being fostered in a loving home.*

The social worker or caring person involved should focus attention on the parent—even in the face of antisocial behavior.

It used to be thought that any kind of parent was better than none at all. However, it is now recognized that if parents repeatedly abuse a child, it is better for the child's physical and mental well-being if he or she is removed from home and placed in a loving, caring environment with foster parents.

Sexual abuse

Child abuse may also be of a sexual nature, and the damage can be done by family members or close family friends. The number of recognized cases has increased because doctors and teachers have learned to recognize the symptoms, but there is growing awareness that this serious problem has existed for many years, even though it may have been hidden inside the family.

Outlook

The problem of child abuse is becoming more widely acknowledged and understood. Whether children who have been physically and emotionally abused grow up to be disturbed depends entirely on how the problem is dealt with and at what stage of development. If the abuse stops and professional help is used to treat the physical and emotional scars, there is no reason why these children should not outgrow the terror of the experience.

See also: Anxiety; Bones; Crying; Depression; Mental illness; Neuroses; Scars

Child development

My one-month-old baby sleeps almost all the time. Is this unusual?

Sleeping patterns vary; some babies are naturally sleepier than others. At around 10 or 12 weeks most sleep through the night and become more wakeful during the day, giving up their midnight feeding. After three months they gradually need less sleep and do not always nap after each meal.

When can I expect my 11-month-old sister to start talking properly?

Probably very soon. Most one-year-olds have about three clear words and babble for the rest of the time in a way that sounds like talking. They understand many words and phrases and will obey simple commands, although they will have learned to shake their heads when they mean no. Children do vary as to the age at which they start to talk, however.

When should a baby start eating solid food?

A baby has no need of solid food until he or she is about three months old. If the baby drinks 2 pints of milk a day and is still hungry (but not overweight), it is a good time to start; more than 2 pints of milk is too much, and the baby needs the concentrated calories of solid food.

My toddler screams and refuses to go to nursery school. How do I make him more independent?

A child has a natural drive toward independence that can't be forced. It could be that your child is too young and feels insecure when you try to leave him with strangers. Once he is secure in the knowledge that a separation doesn't mean losing you forever, he might be happier. Perhaps you could wait until he becomes less dependent.

Human life from birth to age five involves a fascinating series of changes, as helpless infants gradually turn into sociable children who are ready to enter school. What progress can parents expect—and how can they help their children develop healthily and happily?

Children develop at different rates according to their inborn potential, although various factors such as their surroundings and how much attention they receive also influence their progress. The sequence of physical development, and of the acquisition of new skills, does not change, however—some children may be more advanced in some areas and slower in others, but the order in which they develop and learn is the same.

Birth to six months

Feeding: During the first three months of life babies get all the nutrients they need from milk, ideally breast milk. If they are bottle-fed, milk that has been specially prepared for infants should be bought and the formula carefully made up so that the feed is not too concentrated. Formula milk should be used until babies are a year old (using cow's milk before this can lead to an allergy to dairy products). Solid food should be introduced in tiny amounts beginning when the child is three or four months old. By the age of six months, babies will be eating three meals a day with a bottle- or breast-feeding at night. The solids should be finely mashed and the babies given rusks and cut-up vegetables and fruit to handle (see Nutrition).

Crying: Crying is a baby's only method of communication. Parents find out by trial and error why their baby is crying and soon learn to interpret the cries. Small babies usually cry while being undressed or if roughly handled. From six weeks onward almost all babies will stop crying if they are cuddled. By the time they are six months old babies also cry because they are bored or lonely, but they will usually stop when picked up by their mother or father.

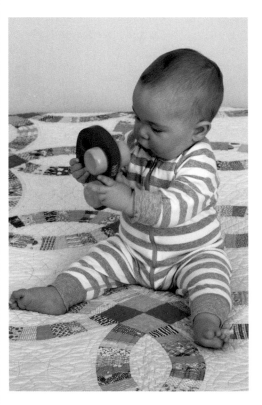

▲ *In the first six months a baby will learn to grasp objects with both hands.*

Physical development: During the first six months, babies learn to support their heads and to roll over by themselves. Eventually they will sit up with a little support, and if their hands are held, they will jump up and down on someone's lap. They also learn to coordinate hand and eye and are able to reach out and grasp objects with both hands. They are likely to cut their first teeth by six months.

Social development and play: From the start babies like to look at a human face, and enjoy the sound of a human voice, above all things. By four weeks they will be making cooing and gurgling noises, and at around six weeks the sounds will be phonetic and infants will "talk back" when spoken to.

The first smiles also come at about six weeks, and babies will smile in response to a smiling face and a human voice. As physical skills develop, they want interesting toys to look at and grasp, and they enjoy being talked to, held, and gently played with.

By the end of their first year, most babies will have cut their two upper front teeth, as well as the two lower ones and one molar.

Relationship with mother: Babies become increasingly attached to their mothers in a highly emotional way, and also become fond of other members of the family and pets. They need their mother's presence constantly, becoming highly disturbed when separated from her, although they will play happily by themselves as long as she is around. They also become unhappy when their mothers show disapproval, but their memory is so short that they are likely to do again the things they were told not to do minutes before—so punishment does no good at this stage.

One to two years

This is the stage between babyhood and childhood, and it can be frustrating for toddlers, who wish to do more than they are physically capable of, and tiring for mothers, since toddlers increasingly demand their own way.

Feeding: Most mothers understand the need for their children to have a good, mixed diet, but sometimes their preoccupation causes

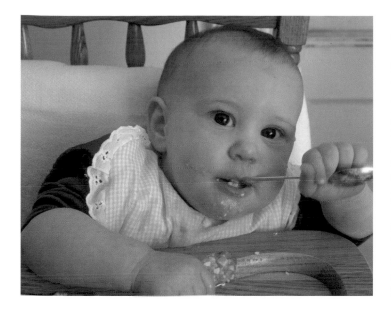

▲ *A baby has a strong will to do things without help—in time this infant will learn to feed himself without too much mess.*

Relationship with mother: By four months babies are usually more relaxed and happy with their mothers than with anyone else. Small babies treat their mother's body as an extension of their own and react with pleasure to the sound of her voice and to her face. They also rely on her for play and entertainment.

Six months to one year

During this period babies start to crawl. They are interested in everything but do not have enough coordination to be gentle with objects. Everything is put into the mouth—this is the way that small babies learn about the world.

Feeding: During this period babies can eat three meals a day at family mealtimes, supplemented by snacks in the morning and afternoon. Their digestive system is able to cope with the food that the family eats as long as it is minced or cut up. However, some mothers prefer to give their babies commercial foods.

Babies will also start to drink from cups and will want to feed themselves. Some babies will still need supplementary bottles, which should be of formula milk until the age of one year.

Crying: At this age babies cry mainly out of frustration and anger at not being able to do the things they want to do, and also from pain if they hurt themselves crawling or attempting to walk. They also cry when left alone—each time a parent leaves for any length of time, it is like a major separation (see Crying).

Social development and play: Babies are less sociable with strangers than they were before and may be suspicious and really frightened of strangers at times. They need more things to play with now.

Physical development: Over these few months babies learn to sit up without support, and then to crawl. They start to pull themselves up to stand, and they may leave out the crawling stage altogether. Once standing, they may move around the room by holding onto furniture. They also become much more practiced at using their hands.

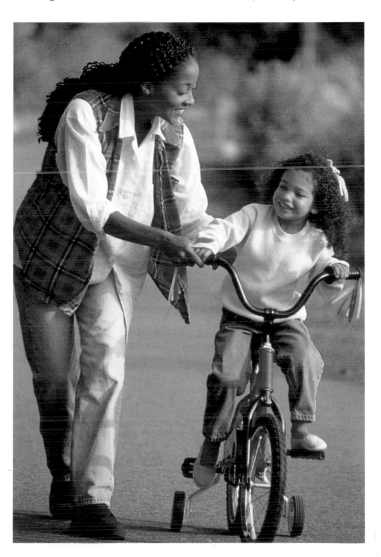

▲ *A child's attempts at learning a new skill are thrilling for a parent. Here a mother teaches her daughter to ride a bicycle.*

Questions and Answers

My one-year-old sister is very shy, even with close family friends. How can I help her?

It is natural for a baby of her age to be shy and dependent on family members. This is a stage that will pass in time, when she is ready to be more sociable. If you try to force her, then her fear of others will increase.

I frequently baby-sit for a two-year-old boy. How do I deal with his temper tantrums?

Tantrums are common in toddlers, and some children have tantrums until they are four years old. It would be more worrying if the child never expressed frustration or bad temper in this way.

Try to avoid frustration: suggest acceptable things to do rather than just saying "don't" when the child does something of which you disapprove. Allow him or her to express aggressive feelings in play. Don't lose your temper; a calm, reassuring attitude will soothe a child. Hold children so that they cannot hurt themselves, and never give in afterward—or they will believe that a tantrum is the way to get what they want.

How can I help my baby niece, who has colic?

Unfortunately, there is no absolute cure for colic. This condition is also called evening colic, because it tends to strike after the late-afternoon or early-evening feeding. It usually starts during the first two weeks of life and rarely lasts longer than nine weeks. It is distressing, for a colicky baby is not comforted even by being cuddled. You may just have to wait until the attacks pass.

My three-year-old son knows lots of words, but he can't make sentences yet. Is this normal?

Most children know about 800 words by age three, and it is at about this time that they start putting together sentences of four or five words.

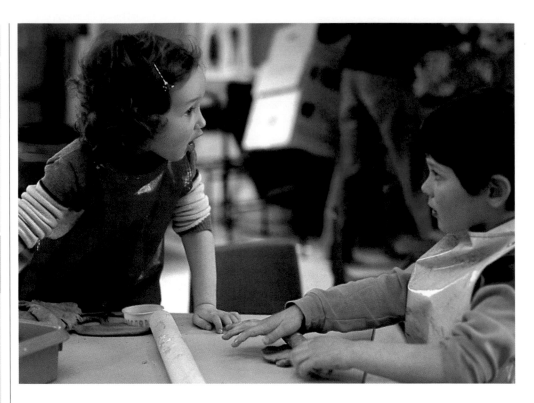

▲ *At nursery school children become used to playing with other children, cooperating and sharing their toys happily.*

feeding problems. Children themselves are a guide to whether they are eating enough of the right things—if they are healthy, growing, and energetic they are getting all the food they need.

Sleeping: Most toddlers of this age have trouble settling down for the night. All will cry when their mother leaves the room. The best solution may be to pop in every five minutes until they settle. Tuck them in with loving words, and say good night again. Children treated like this will not feel lonely and abandoned. They should not be allowed out of the crib, or getting out will become a difficult pattern to break.

Walking: Once toddlers have taken their first few steps, their ability to walk increases rapidly. By 16 months most can toddle well. By 20 months most can run and jump with both feet, but at this age they may prefer to be taken from place to place in a stroller or in their mother's arms.

Talking: The first words babies say are usually the names of loved ones and pets, then the words for favorite foods and drinks, followed by parts of the body, clothes, and everyday articles.

Social development and play: Because of their increased mobility, toddlers are into everything. They are extremely curious and experimental and want to copy what adults or other children do. Their imagination develops, and imaginative play also increases. They are still shy with strangers but may be pushy with other children.

Toilet training: Toilet training cannot begin until toddlers are aware that they have wet or soiled themselves. This can occur anytime between one year and 15 months, and toddlers will begin to indicate to their mother that they have a full diaper. Bladder control follows later—it is far harder for toddlers to "hold on" when they want to urinate. There is no use trying to train them to urinate in the potty if they are still wearing diapers, and they must be allowed the occasional accident. If mothers can remain calm and unemotional, toilet training is likely to be easier. Dirty diapers or pants are not naughty—they are unfortunate.

Relationship with mother: Toddlers are still very reliant on their mothers. They seek more protection and support than ever before, still feel great anxiety over any separation, and resent people who take up their mother's time. At the same time, they are seeking independence, and they resent their smallness and dependence on adults and the power that adults can wield; so they become increasingly negative and assertive, testing their own power against that of the adult world.

Tantrums are common at this age—and for the next year or so. Children are not being willful or naughty but are just reacting to a buildup of frustration that they are too young to control.

Two to five years

This preschool age sees children transformed from dependent babies into social human beings.

Toilet training: Some children will be able to use the potty efficiently by their second year. Others may be as old as three or well into their fourth year before they are completely potty-trained.

Physical development and play: Play is children's equivalent of work. Young children must have space to play and equipment to play with if they are to develop their physical skills. Developing physical skills also fosters self-confidence, independence, and self-reliance and assists emotional development. Fantasy games help social and emotional development.

▼ *By copying his father, this young child is learning to feed himself confidently using chopsticks.*

Social development: Social behavior with other children goes through three recognizable stages, though the transition is gradual and the stages do overlap. During the first stage children are indifferent or aloof with other infants, preferring to play alone. In the next stage they show hostility—they see other children as rivals and may be jealous. In the third stage children become friendly and cooperative, playing happily with other children and sharing toys.

Most children of three or older benefit from time spent at a nursery or child center. The range of equipment available is likely to be far greater there than at home, and a nursery encourages them to learn to do things for themselves that their mothers might do automatically at home. As they get to the stage of friendly cooperation with other children, they learn to give and take.

Relationship with mother: By the end of the first few years children have gone through the stage of being dependent on their mothers and have entered the resistant stage. This will go on into the third year, but as they become more mobile, physically capable, and self-reliant, the relationship should start to settle down. When children realize that their mothers always return after an absence, their separation anxiety decreases, and if they are otherwise confident, they will enjoy the occasional time away from home, perhaps with grandparents. The calmer and happier the first two years are, the more likely children are to become happy and sociable.

See also: **Anxiety; Breast-feeding**

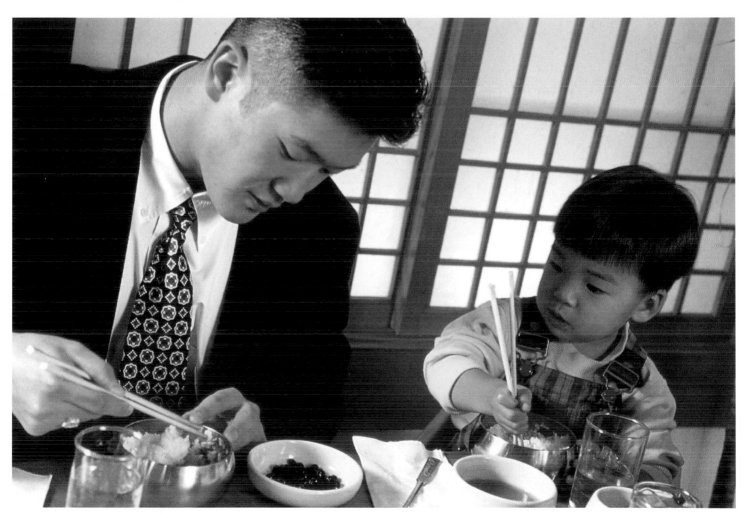

Chinese medicine

For centuries Chinese medicine was considered unscientific and was treated with skepticism in the West. But it has become more widely accepted, and many people use it as an alternative or a complement to Western medicine.

Chinese medicine is based on a philosophy that has evolved over thousands of years. It involves five different therapies: acupuncture, herbs, tui na massage, qigong exercises, and diet. Although each of these therapies can be practiced individually, they all complement each other, and they all have the same underlying principles (see Acupuncture).

The theory

Three main components in Chinese medicine are used in a diagnosis. These are yin and yang, the vital substances, and the five elements. Yin and yang represent the two opposing, but complementary, sides of nature. Everyone has his or her own unique balance of yin and yang, and when yin and yang are in harmony, the body is healthy. When they are out of balance, however, the body becomes ill. The body also contains the vital substances qi (pronounced chi), blood, and body fluids. Qi is an abstract concept that is usually translated as energy or the life force, which the Chinese believe to be the root of all human beings. Although it cannot be seen under a microscope, qi circulates through the body in invisible channels called meridians. If qi becomes deficient or the flow is blocked, this depletes the person's energy and lowers his or her resistance to diseases. The restoration of its flow is vital to regain health.

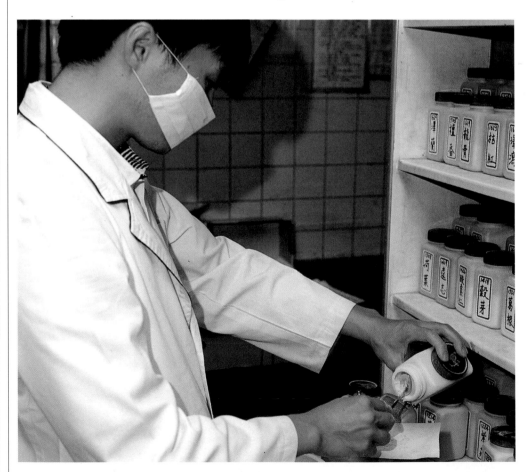

▲ *A pharmacist in a Chinese hospital dispenses traditional herbal medicines from his extensive stock of powdered herbs.*

Questions and Answers

How can I check to see if a practitioner is qualified?

Make sure that he or she is registered with a recognized professional body. Members have to be qualified to belong to the body and will be bound by their code of ethics and code of practice. Qualified practitioners of acupuncture, herbal medicine, and tui na should have trained for at least three or four years.

How do I know which treatment to choose?

Although acupuncture, herbal medicines, and tui na massage can all be used to treat many illnesses, it is usually best to choose the treatment that most appeals to you. Acupuncture is more widely available than other Chinese therapies, and some acupuncturists are also herbalists. Tui na practitioners and qigong teachers are becoming more numerous. You should be able to obtain dietary advice from any Chinese practitioner.

Is it possible to teach myself how to do qigong exercises?

Learn from a qualified teacher. Qigong has proved to be quite dangerous when not done correctly, and people have made themselves ill doing the exercises without the proper training.

Is the Chinese diet vegetarian?

Although much of the diet is based on grains, pulses, and vegetables, the Chinese believe that a healthy diet is one that contains about 2 to 3 oz. (60 to 90 g) of meat a few times a week, to get enough proteins, vitamins, and minerals. If you decide not to eat meat, it is important to eat pulses and grains for protein, and rice, lentils, and fresh vegetables.

Blood is seen as a fluid that nourishes and moisturizes the body while housing the shen or mind-spirit (see Blood). Shen gives us the ability to think, analyze, and discriminate. The state of a person's qi (life force) and blood are dependent on the state of his or her constitution, which is dictated by the strength of the jing essence. Jing is stored in the kidneys and helps us to move through the different stages and cycles of our lives. Jing is inherited, and the amount a person has at birth has to last throughout his or her life.

Fluids called jin ye are the most substantial of all the substances in the body. The jin fluids are light and watery liquids, such as sweat or saliva, that are found near the surface of the body. The ye fluids are heavier and deeper inside the body. If the body fluids do not flow freely, they can obstruct the movement of qi and of blood.

The five elements correspond to everything that makes up the universe—wood, fire, earth, metal, and water. Each is associated with two different internal organs, a yin organ and a yang organ. Water, for example, is associated with the bladder, which is a yang organ, and the kidney, which is a yin organ. The five elements are interconnected; so when one of the organs and its associated element are out of balance, the other elements are also affected.

Making a diagnosis

Chinese medicine is holistic (taking into account both the mind and the body of the patient). This means that the patient's physiological and psychological state will both be considered in making a diagnosis. The practitioner will therefore gather as much information as possible about the patient's symptoms before a physical examination, including looking at the tongue and facial color and taking the pulse. A full diagnosis may take up to two hours.

Acupuncture

This is the best-known treatment, and it is endorsed by the World Health Organization for a wide range of conditions. Acupuncture involves the incision of needles into acupoints on the skin. These acupoints lie along the meridians—the channels along which qi flows. The aim of the needles is to disperse any blockages and bring the qi back into balance. Acupressure is very similar, except that massage techniques rather than needles are used to stimulate the acupoints (see Acupressure). Most acupuncturists use the five elements to discover which organ is the root cause of the condition. The vital substances will also be taken into account, since they may be deficient or may obstruct a particular organ. Moxibustion can be used with acupuncture to speed up the healing process. Heat from herbal charcoal, or from rolled-up cones of the herb moxa, is applied to the end of the acupuncture needle to promote the flow of qi and to restore the body's balance.

Herbal medicine

Chinese herbal medicine can be used for many of the problems that can be treated by acupuncture, although it is known best for its success in treating skin conditions such as eczema and psoriasis.

The practitioner examines the patient first to determine which organs are out of balance and whether the yin and yang energies are in harmony, and then treats the patient accordingly.

Herbal medicines are made from the roots, stems, bark, leaves, seeds, or flowers of many plants, as well as from some mineral and animal products (see Minerals). About 6,000 medicinal items are recorded in the Chinese pharmacopeia (the official list of medicinal

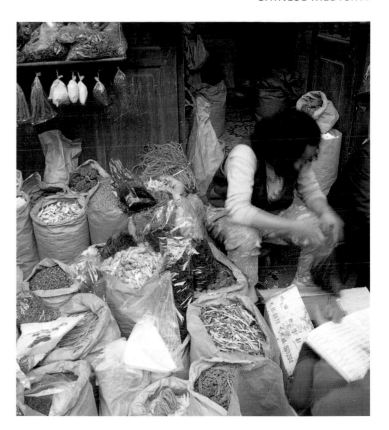

▲ *Traditional medicinal herbs in an East Asian market. In front are sacks of loose plant and animal extracts; small plastic bags of dried herbs can be seen on the shelves.*

substances), and some 400 of them are in common use today. The herbs are prepared in a variety of ways and then made into pills, powders, or tinctures. Some external preparations are also used on the skin as ointments, creams, or herbal plasters. Herbal medicines are usually combinations of herbs known as a prescription. To make the prescription the herbalist carefully blends together a number of herbs, each of which has a specific application. Many of these prescriptions have been created by eminent Chinese herbalists over the past 2,000 years. They differ from Western herbal medicine in that each prescription is a mixture of herbs specially tailored to the patient's needs. The most common way that these herbs are used is in the form of an herbal decoction boiled up from dried herbs—a fresh bag of herbs is boiled up each day. Sometimes the herbalist will use patent herbal pills made by grinding the herbs and mixing them with honey or a paste. These pills are often slightly cheaper than dried herbs and are commonly used for treating deficiencies or acute problems. Powders made of ground-up herbs can be taken directly or mixed with water as a drink. Tinctures are made by extracting the constituents of herbs in a mixture of alcohol and water.

Different tastes

The herbal decoctions or powders vary in taste, and the Chinese have created five main categories to classify them: pungent, sour, sweet, bitter, and salty. There is also a neutral, bland category that has no flavor. The tastes have different effects on the body. The sour, bitter, and salty herbs are more yin and have a downward-moving and internal effect. The sweet, pungent, and neutral herbs are more yang, with an outward-moving and exterior effect.

Questions and Answers

Should I tell my regular doctor I am using Chinese medicine?

You should always tell your doctor if you intend to use any form of Chinese medicine. This is very important if you are having regular treatment or medication. Most doctors do not mind if their patients try these alternatives, especially if traditional medicine has failed to cure a problem. Even if your doctor does not approve, it is still better that he or she should be aware of any treatment you are having.

Is oil used during tui na massage?

Chinese massage does not always require the use of a medium such as oil on the skin. When one is used, it is chosen to suit the particular illness that is being treated. Pure talcum powder and balms like tiger balm may be used, as well as woodlock oil and dong qin gao, which is made from wintergreen mixed with menthol in a petroleum jelly base.

What are Chinese acupuncture needles like?

In the past they were made from bamboo or even stone. Today the needles are usually made from stainless steel, although some practitioners use gold or silver needles. The needles are solid, with a very fine shaft and a sharp point. They come in different lengths, according to which part of the body they are used on. Many acupuncturists prefer single-use disposable needles; others may use an autoclave to sterilize their needles with steam pressure.

Where are Chinese herbs from?

Most of the herbs used in Chinese medicine come from China or Hong Kong. Each herb is harvested, often when it is fully mature. Once collected, the herbs are separated, because different parts of the plant may be used in prescriptions. They are dried and then cut into smaller pieces and exported to the West.

Along with the five tastes, the four energies—hot, warm, cool, and cold temperatures—are also important in deciding which herbs to use. "Temperature" refers to the effect the herbs have on the body rather than whether they themselves are physically hot or cold. Once a prescription has been given, the patient needs to see the practitioner once a month if he or she is suffering from a long-term chronic problem. Acute illnesses such as a cold, cough, or stomach upset require more frequent visits, as herbs may be prescribed for only for a few days.

Qigong exercises

The word "qigong" (pronounced chee-gong) was first used in China in the 1950s to describe a large number of different Chinese exercises. Qigong became very popular in China in the mid-1980s because, as a result of increased freedom, the exercises, which had been closely guarded secrets within families for generations, could now be taught in the open. These exercises are used to strengthen and transform qi energy, and such is their success in China that many myths and legends have grown up around them.

Qigong aims to improve spiritual development in addition to keeping the body healthy. Many practitioners of acupuncture or massage practice qigong to enhance their healing ability. Those who practice regularly over a long period are thought to develop special gifts such as seeing into the future. Although many of the exercises are based on Taoism and Buddhism, qigong does not entail any religious commitment.

Chinese doctors recognized that gentle exercise can stimulate the flow of qi so that it circulates smoothly around the body. Some of the exercises are designed to improve the functioning of different organs in the body, while others help to overcome specific problems. Many exercises have more than one beneficial effect: for example, the "dragon-swimming" exercise has been used extensively by the Chinese to help them lose weight, and it is also thought to strengthen the kidneys, spine, and lower abdomen.

Qigong exercises are all based on three key elements—posture, relaxation, and a focused mind. They can be grouped into four main categories: sitting, standing, moving, and spontaneous moving. Sitting qigong is a form of meditation involving breathing exercises and internal movements such as contracting the anus. Standing qigong involves standing perfectly still in a posture that will help to develop qi. Moving qigong is performed in a gentle, relaxed way

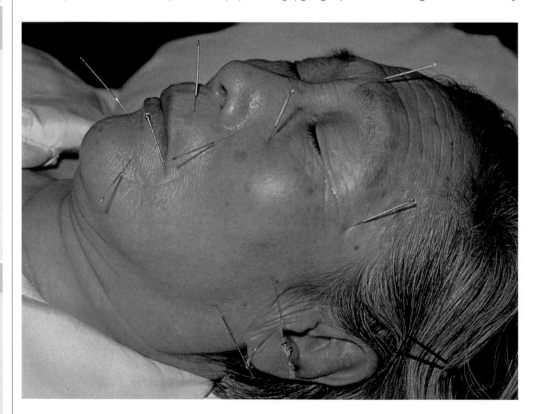

▲ *An elderly patient receives acupuncture treatment for facial palsy, which usually affects one side of the face, making the eyelid and the corner of the mouth droop.*

and requires deep concentration and good posture. Spontaneous moving qigong, the most unusual form of this exercise, involves standing very still until small spontaneous movements occur, such as shaking. It is important to learn qigong from a qualified teacher. Many teachers will teach different types of qigong for different uses, such as for martial arts or for healing. Once the student has learned the exercises, he or she can continue to practice them on a daily basis at home (see Tai Chi).

Tui na

Tui na is a type of therapeutic massage and is one of the oldest forms of Chinese medicine. However, it is still in its infancy in the West, where there are only a relatively small number of qualified practitioners. Tui na literally means "push grab," because this type of massage is usually quite vigorous and fast. It can involve massage techniques such as rolling, pushing, kneading, rubbing, pinching, and pressing. Tui na is beneficial in relieving both acute and chronic joint problems, such as a bad back or a painful knee. It can also help the patient to relax, although it is seldom used just for relaxation. It can be helpful for many of the problems that are treated by acupuncture or herbal medicine. The massage is often carried out at specific acupuncture points on the body or along a meridian line. Once the masseur or masseuse has made a diagnosis, a treatment will be chosen to suit the patient's energy balance. The patient can receive a massage without removing any clothes, although the area to be treated may be covered with a towel or cotton cloth. Treatment usually takes about one hour and will probably need to be repeated frequently at first, being reduced gradually as the condition improves. There are various techniques that can be used for self-massage, but these are best taught by a qualified practitioner.

Chinese dietary therapy

Chinese dietary therapy is based on eating the correct proportion of different types of food, also taking into account the temperature,

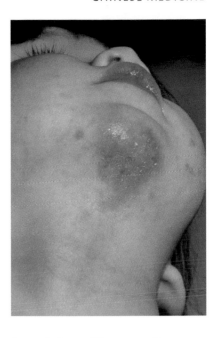

▶ *Eczema—a red, oozing rash that itches —is a condition that often responds well to treatment with Chinese herbal medicine.*

taste, and quantity of the food, and how and when it is eaten. The Chinese believe that a good diet is important not just for physical well-being but also for mental health, because everything we eat ultimately becomes one of the vital substances, such as qi, blood, or body fluids. If one of the digestive organs is not functioning properly, fatigue, poor skin, and poor hair condition, as well as many digestive disorders, can result. Poor function can also affect concentration and memory. A healthful Chinese diet will contain more grains, fruit, and vegetables, and less meat, sugar, and fat than most Western diets. The diet should be made up of 40 to 60 percent grains and pulses, 20 to 30 percent fruit and vegetables, and about 10 to 15 percent meat, fat, dairy products, and seafood.

The Chinese class all food as either hot, warm, neutral, cool, or cold. This categorization refers to the warming or cooling effect the food has on the body, rather than whether the food itself is physically hot or cold. It is generally considered best to eat foods that are neither too hot nor too cold, such as rice, which is considered to be the most nourishing grain for this reason. Food should also be cooked, as raw food is "cold" and therefore harder to digest.

How and where food is eaten is important too, since people should be in a relaxed state when eating so that digestion can work properly. Food needs to be eaten at regular intervals and should be well chewed to aid the digestive process.

Dietary rules

It is thought that liquids should not be drunk at mealtimes, as this interferes with digestion. It is also advisable to stop eating when three quarters full so that the stomach has time to empty before the next meal. The Chinese believe that the correct diet will help to maintain good health in a patient after he or she has undergone treatment through acupuncture, herbal medicine, or massage. Correct diet is also thought to help if used alongside any of the other Chinese therapies (see Alternative Medicine; Diet).

Professional help

As with all Chinese medicine, it is important to go to a fully trained practitioner for treatment. One of the best ways of finding a practitioner is by personal recommendation; alternatively, find someone through one of the various professional bodies.

See also: Diagnosis; Eczema; Exercise; Herbs and herbalism; Massage; Psoriasis; Skin and skin diseases; Temperature

---

Common illnesses that can be helped by Chinese medicine

Acupuncture, herbal medicine, and tui na can be used alongside qigong and Chinese dietary therapy to treat a wide variety of illnesses, including the following.

Breathing problems: asthma, coughs, bronchitis, hay fever

Circulatory problems: angina, high and low blood pressure, palpitations, poor circulation, varicose veins

Digestive complaints: gallstones, gastritis, indigestion, nausea, stomach ulcers, constipation, diarrhea

Emotional conditions: anxiety, depression, eating disorders, panic attacks

Gynecological problems: heavy periods, menopausal problems, premenstrual syndrome, postnatal depression, vaginal discharge

Chiropractic

Questions and Answers

What is the difference between an osteopath and a chiropractor?

They offer similar treatments, but compared with an osteopath a chiropractor uses manipulation as the main form of treatment, as opposed to soft-tissue or massage techniques. Some chiropractors will also offer dietary advice. Osteopaths in the United States are medically qualified and are usually consulted primarily for their medical expertise.

Are chiropractors actually medically qualified?

No, but the chiropractic preclinical education standards are now recognized to be equal to those of medicine. U.S. students must have credits from at least two years of a bachelor's degree course before they can start chiropractic training. They study chiropractic techniques for four to five years full-time as well as required medical sciences.

Is chiropractic treatment painful?

This depends on your sensitivity, your type of problem, and the way in which individual chiropractors make adjustments. Generally, the more painful your condition, the more likely you are to experience some discomfort. Many patients feel tired after treatment, and stiffness or soreness may occur for a few days afterward. Pain could increase as tight muscles readjust, but this is unlikely. If you are worried, contact your chiropractor.

How do I find a good chiropractor?

Your doctor can refer you to a fully qualified, registered chiropractor; otherwise a chiropractic association will usually supply a list of registered chiropractors. The initials DC after a qualified chiropractor's name stand for doctor of chiropractic.

Chiropractors diagnose joint conditions and use manipulative techniques to improve joint function and to relieve pain and muscle spasm. Chiropractic is primarily used in the treatment of back pain.

Manipulating the spine is one of the oldest healing therapies in the world (see Manipulation). A 5th-century votive relief excavated from the Aesculapian hospital in Piraeus, Greece, shows the healer Aesculapius manipulating the upper thoracic spine (see Spinal Cord). However, by the 19th century, medicine was increasingly starting to involve only scientifically proved treatments.

In America most medical progress was being made on the East Coast; elsewhere, in rural areas in particular, where there were fewer trained doctors, there was dissatisfaction with medical methods. This encouraged a general interest in natural healing, including bone-setting (see Bones). It was not until September 1885, however, that chiropractic was "discovered," when the healer Daniel David Palmer (1845–1913) treated a caretaker, Harvey Lillard, for a 17-year-old injury. Lillard had been bent over his work when he felt something give in his back. At almost the same time he lost his hearing. Palmer repositioned the vertebra that had moved, Lillard's hearing allegedly improved, and chiropractic began.

▲ *Chiropractic is based on the theory that many of the physical complaints of the human body can be traced to an incorrect alignment of the spine.*

Early theories

Two decades earlier the founder of osteopathy, Andrew Taylor Still (1828–1917), had developed the theory that many ailments stem from distortions or malfunctions in the structure of the body (see Osteopathy). Although the theories are similar, Palmer's first spinal adjustment convinced him that the basis of all disease lay in the spine, because the human nervous system was affected if the vertebrae of the spine were misaligned (see Nervous System). Palmer talked to doctors and taught himself anatomy and physiology, and then developed his own system of treatment.

Palmer came up against much opposition from the established medical profession and in 1906 was jailed for three months for practicing without a medical license. Meanwhile his son, Bartlett Joshua Palmer (1882–1961), took over the Palmer Infirmary and Chiropractic Institute—and it was not long before he had turned the institute into a profitable concern.

Shortly after Daniel's release, father and son parted company. Daniel Palmer spent the next seven years attempting to establish schools as he traveled through the Indian Territory, California, Oregon, and Canada. The same year that he died, Kansas became the first state to license chiropractors. Bartlett Joshua continued to work at the school, influencing the chiropractic profession until his death in 1961. He introduced X-ray analysis, and together with other early chiropractors used this to pioneer new techniques and methods of study. Bartlett Joshua insisted on a purist approach and opposed those who incorporated other methods of natural healing.

In the 1930s Bartlett Joshua developed the hole-in-one technique, believing that if the top two vertebrae were aligned, the full health of the patient could be achieved. This policy was revised in 1958 in accordance with the teachings of other major chiropractic colleges in the country.

In 1974, two years after Congress had voted to make chiropractic available under Medicare, chiropractic became legal throughout the United States. In the same year, the Wisconsin Workers Compensation Board identified chiropractic as the most economic form of treatment for back pain, and studies repeated in the other states drew the same conclusion (see Back and Backache).

Today chiropractic has emerged as a major form of treatment for back pain, with an estimated one in 15 Americans consulting a chiropractor at least once a year.

How it works

The basic principle of chiropractic is that the architecture of a healthy spine is designed to assist normal body functioning. Chiropractors manipulate joints that have been subjected to abnormal pressures, which have damaged their function. The chiropractor's aim is to restore normal joint functioning and thereby improve overall health.

All of the body's joints contain cells called mechanoceptors, which register movement. Stimulating these mechanoceptors produces pain-relieving hormones, or endorphins; this result is one of the reasons why soft-tissue massage around the joints may also be effective.

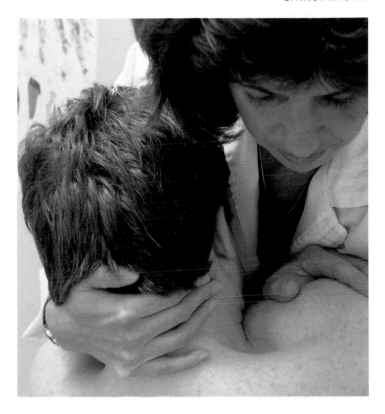

▲ *A chiropractor attempts to correct this man's nerve function by manipulating the spinal column.*

Conditions the chiropractor can treat

The following common conditions may be helped or relieved by chiropractic treatment:
Neck pain caused by strain on posterior joints and ligaments
Tension headaches due to problems in the upper cervical spine and muscle spasm
All back pain, except when there is a serious underlying pathological cause or where nerve roots are so trapped that surgical decompression is necessary
Thoracic spine pain involving the costovertebral joints
Lower back pain due to strain on facet joints, sacroiliac, and ligaments, causing associated muscle spasm and referred pain
Occasionally disk herniation or an abnormally protruding disk
Irritation of nerve roots—including cramplike leg pain—caused by lateral spinal canal stenosis, the narrowing of the canal carrying the spinal cord
Problems in peripheral joints, such as rotator cuff tendinitis and shoulder capsulitis (both are types of shoulder inflammation), tennis elbow, and carpal tunnel syndrome—numbness, tingling, and pain in the thumb, index, and middle fingers
Problems in hand and foot joints
Sprained knee ligaments and minor meniscal tears
Ankle injuries

When to see a chiropractor

Treatment is suitable for people of all ages, although only a specialist should manipulate babies, and it is essential that pregnant women inform the chiropractor of their condition before the consultation. A few chiropractors specialize in the treatment of animals.

Since chiropractors aim to restore the correct functioning of the joints, any person with an appropriate joint problem is likely to benefit. Occasionally organic illnesses have been successfully treated, but most people go to a chiropractor to relieve back pain, usually in the lower back. Mild backaches tend to disappear within weeks, in which case they do not need treatment. But expert advice should be sought after a sudden sprain, strain, or heavy fall, or if the pain continues or recurs (see Sprains; Tendons).

The next most common problem area is the neck (see Neck). Incorrect posture and tension can cause the neck muscles to tighten, and this may refer pain to other areas of the body, particularly the shoulders and arms (see Muscles). Whiplash can also be helped by chiropractic treatment, as can many sports injuries, such as sprained joints or ligaments, strained muscles, and damaged intervertebral disks (see Sports Injury). Chiropractic may also reduce pain caused by the aftereffects of injury or surgery when traditional methods of treatment have failed.

What happens in a consultation

On a first visit, the chiropractor will ask about the patient's medical history and whether he or she is taking prescribed drugs. The chiropractor will also want details of any injuries. Questions may sometimes be asked about the patient's lifestyle, such as working and eating habits. This information is treated as confidential. A thorough physical examination will follow, during which the

Questions and Answers

How long does a course of chiropractic treatment last?

The number and frequency of treatments depend on your needs and the chiropractor's approach. Chronic conditions generally take longer to treat than recent, acute problems. Each time you visit, the chiropractor will reassess your condition. Most patients receive between four and 12 treatments. Patients with conditions that are not completely curable may need to return at regular, longer intervals for improvements to be maintained.

What causes the popping when the chiropractor adjusts my spine?

Often a slight click is heard as an adjustment is made. Patients usually assume that this is the noise made by a vertebra going back into place. But the only joints that can move at all during spinal adjustment are the facet joints that link the vertebrae. The noise is heard because the joint surfaces are being forced apart during manipulation. This alters the balance of pressure from the synovial fluid surrounding each joint. The "pop" is similar in principle to cracking the knuckles.

Is chiropractic treatment safe?

No medical treatment can be guaranteed to be entirely safe, but complications arising from chiropractic treatment are minimal, especially when X rays are used to prevent misdiagnosis. Doctors of chiropractic receive academic and clinical training, are licensed by law to provide diagnostic and therapeutic services, and refer patients to other health care practitioners when appropriate.

In the unlikely event of an accident, most chiropractic associations have procedures for handling complaints. Manipulation should not be carried out in cases of acute arthritis, malignant tumors, tuberculosis, fractures, and some bone diseases, and should rarely be used in cases of prolapsed disks. All chiropractors should adhere to safety guidelines.

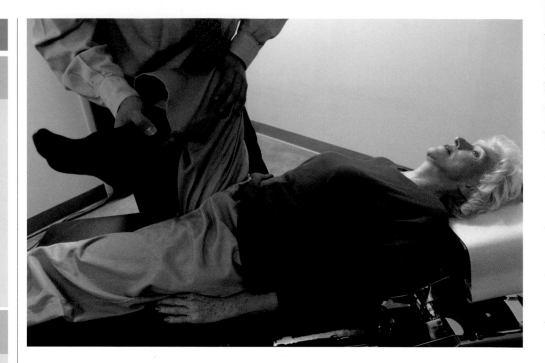

▲ *Patients often lie on a special couch as they are treated by the chiropractor.*

patient is asked to take off outer garments and go through a series of maneuvers. During the exercises, the chiropractor assesses posture, leg length, and mobility. The chiropractor also uses palpation, or analysis by touch, at various times to enable himself or herself to judge skin and muscle tone and the condition of ligaments and bones. A light rubber hammer is used to test leg and arm reflexes (see Reflexes). Healthy reflexes mean that clear messages are being sent from an area to the spinal cord via the nervous system, and that the area is free from disturbance. Other tests may be chosen also, depending on the type of problem presented. If necessary, X rays may be taken (see X Rays).

Treatment is sometimes given at the end of the first consultation with the chiropractor, but not if X-ray results are required. Occasionally the chiropractor decides that a condition is unsuitable for treatment, and he or she refers the patient back to the doctor. Chiropractors are trained to make a diagnosis, but if a condition is particularly painful or chronic, it is advisable to see a doctor before visiting a chiropractor.

Treatment

Many patients who seek treatment for back pain have developed postural problems. In order to maintain balance, the body compensates for any postural distortion, and it does this by causing one or more counterdistortions elsewhere in the spine or pelvis. This is the main reason why treatment may involve areas other than the site of pain and why a number of visits may be necessary.

Treatment includes soft-tissue work along with manipulation. Patients are usually asked to lie on a special couch, but they may be asked to sit, kneel, or stand. The two main types of manipulation are direct adjustment and toggle recoil. Direct adjustment involves a rapid, shallow movement that is sometimes accompanied by a "pop." Any pain is usually from inflamed tissues rather than caused by the adjustment (see Inflammation). Toggle recoil involves carefully positioning the patient before performing a split-second thrusting movement. This is said to induce relaxation around the joint tissues and to allow the joint to return to normal mobility and function. Back, leg, or arm joints may be manipulated, and sometimes the skull and face are manipulated. Some chiropractors offer mechanical means of pain relief, such as ultrasound, for short periods only. In the United States, members of the American Chiropractic Association (ACA) incorporate other therapies into their treatment, placing emphasis on nutrition and vitamin and mineral supplements.

See also: Joints; Knee; Ligaments; Massage; Pelvis; Physical therapy; Posture; Shoulder; Skeleton; Tennis elbow; Whiplash Injury

Cholera

Questions and Answers

Will I need a cholera vaccination to go on vacation to India, and will I need a certificate of proof?

Cholera vaccinations are voluntary in many countries but are strongly recommended in places such as India. People traveling from India to certain other countries will also need an International Certificate of Vaccination. The best thing to do is to get details of all vaccinations needed from your travel agent, or directly from the embassy of the country you intend to visit.

Can poor housing and overcrowding cause cholera?

Cholera remains a threat to all communities where sanitation and hygiene standards are poor. The disease is not regularly found in the United States, because there is no population of carriers (people who carry the bacteria but show no symptoms). But with foreign travel becoming more widespread, it is easier for an unidentified carrier to enter a city and start an outbreak. It is only because water supplies are so carefully controlled, and because of the high standard of personal hygiene, that cholera does not affect the United States.

Why does cholera appear after some form of natural disaster, such as an earthquake?

Cholera breaks out whenever drinking and cooking water have been contaminated by infected excreta. In earthquake areas drainage pipes for sewage water may crack and leak into the wells or rivers that provide clean water. Where large numbers of people are living and cooking together in temporary camps, the disposal of excreta may be poor and hygiene virtually impossible, owing to lack of water. A cholera epidemic can also occur as a result of food contamination, when flies feed off sewage and then settle on food.

Cholera is an acute bacterial infection that causes severe diarrhea and vomiting. It is spread in water contaminated by human feces and vomit, and it usually occurs only in areas where hygiene and sanitation are poor.

Cholera is a serious, highly infectious, and often fatal bacterial infection of the intestine. It causes profuse watery diarrhea and vomiting, which lead to death through a massive dehydration of the body tissues.

Causes

The bacterium that causes cholera is *Vibrio cholerae*, known as the comma bacillus—a reference to its short, commalike shape. It can be transmitted either by people infected with cholera or by those who have survived the disease. The most common method of transmission is that an infected person fouls a freshwater supply with his or her excreta and vomit (see Infection and Infectious Diseases).

Symptoms

The incubation period lasts from between 12 hours and six days. About 90 percent of people infected show symptoms; the remainder suffer few or no ill effects. The disease starts with uncontrollable diarrhea, nausea, and massive dehydration, followed by raging thirst. The kidneys or heart may fail, and patients may die at this stage, but in many cases their condition improves. If the damage to the heart or kidneys is too severe, however, the disease is fatal.

Treatment

Prompt medical treatment can reduce the mortality rate from 50 percent to 1 percent, and rehydration is the most important element. Although rehydration is usually achieved with intravenous fluids, it can be done orally. When treatment is delayed, the death rate rises. People with mild cases recover spontaneously, but in serious cases of cholera the outlook depends on how much fluid is lost and what medical treatment is received.

See also: **Bacteria; Diarrhea**

Prevention
BEFORE ENTERING A CHOLERA AREA
Be vaccinated: protection lasts up to a year.
Take tetracycline antibiotics for further protection if infection is likely.
IN A CHOLERA AREA
Isolate all suspected victims.
Burn all contaminated items.
Identify and treat asymptomatic carriers.
Boil all water, and avoid uncooked food that may have been contaminated.
Protect food from insects.
Wash hands after using the toilet and before handling food.
Carefully dispose of all sewage.

WHERE CHOLERA VACCINATION IS NECESSARY

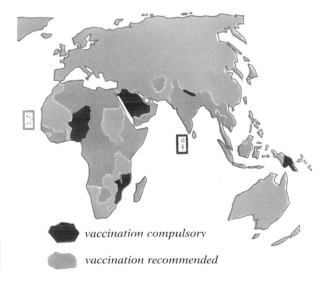

vaccination compulsory

vaccination recommended

Cholesterol

A certain amount of cholesterol is essential to health, but too much can contribute to artery disease and heart attacks. Careful attention to diet and lifestyle will help to avoid potential problems.

Will a low-cholesterol diet help me avoid getting heart disease?

It might, but only when combined with other measures, such as quitting smoking (if you smoke), which causes the arteries to contract and so makes them more likely to clog. Other precautionary measures are controlling your weight, exercising regularly, and avoiding stress whenever possible.

Does a high level of blood cholesterol run in families? Several of my relations have had heart attacks. Is there any connection?

Yes, there are some well-known medical conditions in which abnormalities of the fats and cholesterol in the blood are inherited. People thus affected may need intensive treatment with both diet and drugs.

My son has always been teased about being fat. Does this mean he has a high blood cholesterol level?

Not necessarily. People who are very overweight consume more food than they need, storing the excess food energy in the form of fat. Their blood cholesterol, however, depends largely on the makeup of their diet, and your son may also be eating the wrong kinds of foods. Try to get him to cut out fast food, ice cream, cake, and candy, but remember that losing weight too quickly or eating too little could damage his health.

Are there any danger signs of a high cholesterol level?

Most people with yellowish deposits of cholesterol around the eyes, called xanthelasma, do not have raised blood cholesterol levels, but a check is justified. When this condition is present in young people, the cholesterol levels should always be checked.

Cholesterol is a fatty or oily substance that normally forms part of the wall around each cell in the body. It is also a basic building block of the steroid hormones, a major group of the body's chemical messengers. However, when cholesterol becomes lodged in the arterial walls, it can contribute to the condition called atherosclerosis, or hardening of the arteries, which causes heart attacks and strokes—a major cause of death in the Western world. The body usually makes sufficient cholesterol, but levels may be increased by extra amounts of animal fats and eggs in the diet (see Fats).

People at risk

A number of factors contribute to the risk of arterial or heart disease. Smoking and a family history of these conditions are as important as the level of cholesterol in the blood. People in the United States get about 40 percent of their food energy from fats. Surveys of other groups of people who traditionally eat a less fatty diet suggest that if this figure were reduced to below 30 percent, cholesterol levels would probably be lowered. Such a reduction could be achieved by replacing fats with carbohydrates (starchy foods such as bread, potatoes, and rice). Also, fats of animal origin—the so-called saturated fats—seem to increase cholesterol levels, whereas unsaturated fats, such as sunflower, safflower, and corn oil, do not.

What happens in the body

Only a quarter of the cholesterol that circulates in the blood comes directly from the digestive tract, where it has been absorbed from food. Some of the circulating cholesterol returns to the liver, where it is broken down and secreted as bile by the gallbladder. Any excess may enter the arterial walls.

The body binds cholesterol with protein to form lipoproteins, of which there are two forms: a low-density (or lightweight) form called LDL and a heavy-density form called HDL. Relative to HDL, LDL is lightweight because it contains more fat; therefore, LDL floats. LDL deposits cholesterol in the walls of arteries, and can thus be regarded as the bad lipoprotein. HDL, on the other hand, seems to operate in reverse by mopping up loose cholesterol from the arteries and elsewhere in the body and carrying it back to the liver, where it is broken down in the bile and excreted. A greater proportion of HDL in the blood has beneficial effects. The only known way to increase HDL is through exercise. Although much research is being carried out into HDL and LDL, how they work is not yet known. However, it is clear that lowering the cholesterol level helps prevent heart attacks.

Altering the diet

Most experts agree that a sensible diet can help prevent heart attacks. Consumption of sugar, in many commercially made foods, should be reduced and consumption of poultry, fish, and vegetable protein increased. Carbohydrates are best eaten as bread, potatoes, rice, and beans. Red meat should be eaten only once every few days, and no more than four eggs per week should be eaten. Fats should be half of vegetable (polyunsaturated fats) and half of animal origin.

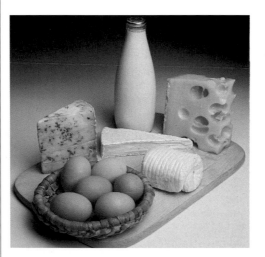

▲ *These foods contain large amounts of fat and should be eaten in moderation.*

See also: **Arteries and artery disease; Diet; Dieting; Heart attack; Hormones; Protein**

Chorionic villus sampling

My doctor says I should have a chorionic villus sample taken. If it shows something wrong, will the doctors be able to cure it?

Unfortunately not. Like all screening procedures, chorionic villus sampling can only point out a possible problem with an unborn baby. If the test does show that the baby has a problem, you will have a choice between continuing with the pregnancy, knowing what the outcome will be, and having an abortion. Medical treatment cannot usually begin until after the birth. Remember also that a negative result does not guarantee a perfect baby, because there are defects, such as heart conditions, that the test cannot pick up.

Can I refuse to have a chorionic villus sample done if the hospital offers me one, or can my doctor insist that I have it?

You cannot be forced to have any test during pregnancy. Your doctor may offer you a variety of tests that he or she feels would provide useful information, but you do not have to take them.
   It may, however, help you to discuss the matter with a counselor before making your final decision.

I have three daughters and have found that I am pregnant again. My husband desperately wants a son this time. Would chorionic villus sampling determine the sex of the baby? My husband would be so disappointed if it is a girl that I would consider an abortion.

Chorionic villus sampling is a serious medical procedure that is intended to discover fetal abnormalities at an early stage. No doctor would agree to perform the procedure simply to learn the sex of your unborn child. Perhaps you and your husband should consider couples counseling or marriage guidance.

This modern, painless diagnostic technique can be used in the very earliest stages of pregnancy, between weeks 10 and 11, to detect a variety of possible disorders in a developing fetus.

Chorionic villus sampling (CVS) is a technique for obtaining information about an unborn baby that can be performed as early as 10 weeks after fertilization. Results are ready within a few days. This gives it an advantage over the similar technique of amniocentesis (in which a sample of the amniotic fluid surrounding the fetus is removed by means of a syringe for testing). Amniocentesis can be performed only from the 16th week after fertilization and takes several weeks to produce results.

Why it is done

Chorionic villus sampling is used to test for a variety of chromosomal, metabolic, and genetic abnormalities, including Down syndrome, cystic fibrosis, spina bifida, thalassemia, and Tay-Sachs disease, and sex-linked abnormalities such as Duchenne muscular dystrophy and some forms of hemophilia. Unlike amniocentesis, it cannot detect neural tube defects. The test is generally offered to older pregnant women, because the procedure carries some risks and the likelihood of chromosomal abnormalities is higher in older mothers. It may also be offered to younger women

▼ *When taking a villi sample through the abdominal wall, the doctor holds an ultrasound scanner on the abdomen, which gives a picture of the inside of the uterus on the screen.*

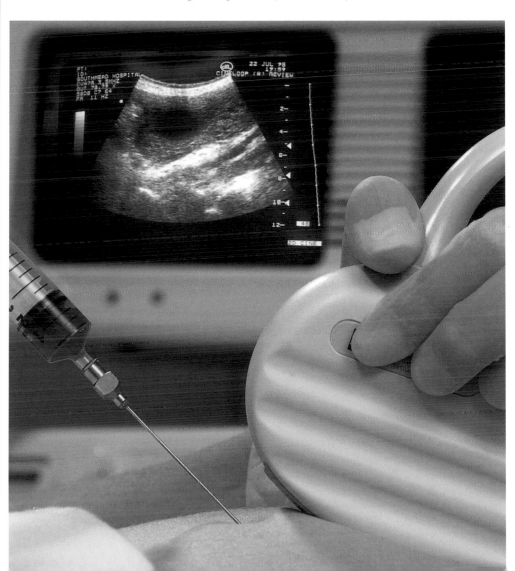

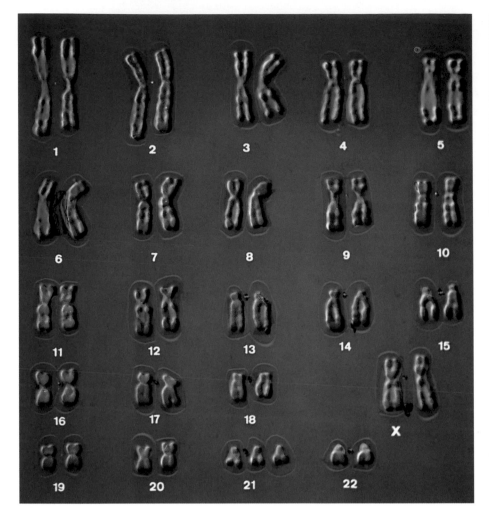

1 2 3 4 5

6 7 8 9 10

11 12 13 14 15

16 17 18 X

19 20 21 22

◄ *In the pairing of chromosomes in a girl with Down syndrome, the 21st set has an extra chromosome, which produces the condition. This is one of the defects that can be detected by analyzing a chorionic villus sample.*

The main advantage of this procedure over amniocentesis is that if any abnormalities are found, the mother will be aware of them much earlier. For many women it is easier to decide on termination early in the pregnancy rather than at around 20 weeks, as happens with the amniocentesis procedure.

One of the reasons CVS has not replaced amniocentesis is that the risk of miscarriage is slightly higher. The miscarriage rate for CVS, about 1 percent, is the same as for amniocentesis, but because the background spontaneous miscarriage rate at 10 weeks is higher, the overall rate for chorionic villus sampling is 2 to 3 percent. In some cases, even when miscarriage does not occur, the wall of the uterus is damaged, causing complications at birth. Chorionic villus sampling may cause limb deformities in 0.03 to 0.1 percent of cases. Rarely, nutritional and growth problems occur later in the pregnancy (see Miscarriage).

at risk, either because of their family history or because of a previous pregnancy with chromosomal abnormalities.

Early in a pregnancy the embryo forms two parts—one becomes the fetus and the other the placenta, which carries nourishment to the growing fetus. The part that forms the placenta starts out as fingerlike chorionic villi (literally, shaggy hairs). They burrow into the wall of the uterus, where they come into contact with the mother's blood vessels. The placenta starts to form after 12 weeks, and a sample of villi is removed for testing before then. The tests can be carried out between 10 and 11 weeks. Because the villi are formed by division of the fertilized egg, they have the same chromosomes, including any genetic abnormality, as the embryo. If the villi test positive for chromosomal abnormalities, so will the embryo.

How the test is done
The test is carried out in the hospital under a local anesthetic. If a women is anxious, she may be given a sedative before the test. A small sample of the chorionic villi is obtained by one of two methods: either a fine, flexible tube is passed through the vagina and the cervix (the neck of the uterus) and guided to the villi by means of an ultrasound scanner, where a sample of the villi is sucked out by a syringe; or a needle is passed through the abdominal wall, as in amniocentesis, using ultrasound to locate the villi. The procedure is slightly uncomfortable, but not painful, and takes about one hour. The cells from the villi are then cultured and chromosome analysis is performed.

Who is offered the test
If a doctor feels that an expectant mother is at significant risk of carrying a fetus with one of the conditions that chorionic villus sampling can detect—perhaps an earlier blood test has given cause for concern—he or she may offer a CVS. The risks and benefits will be explained, and the woman will be made aware of the possibility of terminating the pregnancy if the fetus is found to be affected.

Most hospitals offer counseling, which should be given before the decision to have the test and again afterward if the sample shows some abnormality. If termination is legal where she lives, the expectant mother will be offered this option. Although for some women termination is out of the question for religious or other reasons, knowing in advance that their baby is going to be handicapped helps them to prepare before the birth so that they are ready to cope both mentally and practically when the baby is born.

See also: **Amniocentesis; Birth defects; Spina bifida**

Chronic fatigue syndrome

Chronic fatigue syndrome (CFS) has come to be commonly recognized by the medical profession only in recent years. However, sufferers from the syndrome have been only too aware of the condition for some time.

The main characteristic of chronic fatigue syndrome is continual physical tiredness, which may be as severe as incapacitating exhaustion. There is usually also mental tiredness. Many people with CFS were formerly said to have myalgic encephalomyelitis (ME), but this term has now been abandoned, as encephalomyelitis is inflammation of the brain and spinal cord, which is not a feature of CFS. CFS is also known as postviral fatigue syndrome, as it often follows viral infections.

I first read about chronic fatigue syndrome only a few years ago. Is this a completely new disease?

It has been known for a long time that viral infections are often followed by a period of depression and tiredness. This is particularly noticeable in conditions such as mononucleosis. Doctors have known about chronic fatigue syndrome for some time, but there was a lot of publicity about it in the early 1980s, and the diagnosis has been more common since then.

I have heard people refer to the "yuppie syndrome." Is this another term for chronic fatigue syndrome?

Yes. The term "yuppie syndrome" arose for three main reasons: it mostly affects people below the age of 40, it often affects those who are exhausted by a stressful lifestyle, and it was named around the same time as so-called yuppies (young urban professionals) were.

My brother has been diagnosed as suffering from chronic fatigue syndrome. My father thinks that he's just lazy. Could my brother's condition be all psychological?

Certain psychological states mimic CFS outwardly, but if a doctor has diagnosed CFS in your brother, his condition will be mainly physical. Nevertheless, CFS does cause some psychological depression. Support from those near him, such as his family and close friends, will help.

A friend told me that there was an CFS epidemic at her sister's office. Do such epidemics really happen?

Most of the time a single individual is affected by CFS, but epidemics sometimes do occur in hospitals, schools, offices, and factories, where people spend a lot of time together.

Symptoms

The feeling of physical tiredness varies in degree and may be accompanied by aching muscles. Physical exercise often makes the symptoms worse. The mental tiredness may be associated with emotional disturbances, which arise either from the condition itself or from the frustration sufferers can feel because of the exhaustion. The general tiredness can have drastic effects on sufferers' lifestyles. They are often unable to work or take part in social activities for some considerable time. Some people are completely incapacitated for all practical purposes.

Causes

Beyond the fact that CFS follows viral infections, and often a series of infections, little is known about its real causes. There is some evidence that infections of the digestive system, which later move into the rest of the body, may be involved. But other viruses—such as those that cause influenza, mononucleosis, and rubella (German measles)—may also cause the conditions. Recent research shows that some continuous viral infection is involved in both cases, with improvement occurring when antibodies to the virus disappear from the bloodstream.

Recovery

There are no specific treatments for CFS other than time and plenty of rest. Because of the depression that the condition causes, which can in itself hinder recovery, it is particularly important that the mind, as well as the body, is cared for and nurtured. A generally healthy diet and lifestyle can help speed recovery, as can a positive mental attitude.

People with CFS recover, and the condition is never fatal. However, recovery may take months, and this fact can be very dispiriting for the sufferer, especially if a seeming recovery then falters for a while. Most cases of CFS involve a strong psychological element, and some are wholly psychological in origin. Recent studies have shown that, regardless of the causation, cognitive behavior therapy seems to offer better hope for early recovery than any other form of treatment.

See also: **Blood; Depression; Diet; Digestive system; Influenza; Lethargy; Psychology; Rubella; Viruses**

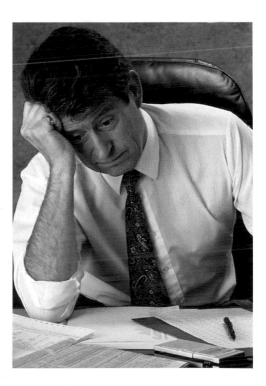

▲ *Inability to concentrate and excessive tiredness after only a short time at work are symptoms of chronic fatigue syndrome.*

Chronic obstructive pulmonary disease

Chronic obstructive pulmonary disease interferes with the flow of air from the atmosphere to the bloodstream, which transports oxygen to the body tissues. When the interference is continuous and of long duration, it is very dangerous.

Chronic obstructive pulmonary disease (COPD) refers to a persistent inflammation of the air tubes of the lungs, or to the lung disease emphysema or, more often, to a combination of both conditions. In the early stages, chronic bronchitis is a fairly mild disease. However, with time and continued abuse of the lungs by smoking cigarettes, it is likely to progress to the condition known as COPD.

How airway obstruction occurs

The term "obstruction" is used here to mean any interference with the passage of oxygen from the atmosphere to the blood. The obstruction to airflow is not just a narrowing of air tubes (bronchi) by inflammatory swelling, sputum (phlegm), and thickening of the walls. In addition, the long-term infection of the small airways causes the weakening and eventual breakdown of large numbers of tiny air sacs in the lungs, resulting in a smaller number of larger air spaces. The total surface area available for oxygen transfer to the blood is therefore greatly reduced, so that the affected person becomes short of oxygen. This breakdown of lung tissue is called emphysema.

As well as cutting down the amount of oxygen that can get into the blood, emphysema results in a loss of lung elasticity and the collapse of the small air passages in the lungs. Normal expiration is a passive process caused by lung elasticity, so when this is lost, expiration becomes more difficult. Some patients with this problem have to purse their lips when breathing out to slow down their exhalation at the mouth so that they can maintain enough pressure in their lungs to keep the airway partly open (see Lung and Lung Diseases).

Causes

COPD is caused by cigarette smoking. Other factors are much less important but may contribute to its development. They include a family history of COPD with a possible genetic element, inhaling other people's cigarette smoke (secondary smoking), inhalation of polluted air in industrial settings and in areas of high automobile density, and a history of childhood chest

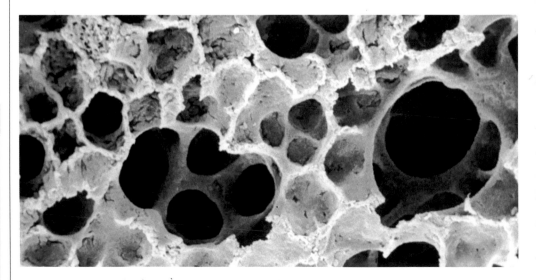

▲ *This falsely colored electron micrograph scan shows the dark air sacs in a normal lung, which can become damaged and restricted in the lungs of victims of COPD.*

Questions and Answers

My father is often breathless and can look blue around the mouth. Our doctor has told him that he has COPD. What does this mean?

Chronic obstructive pulmonary disease. Pulmonary disease is lung disease. "Chronic" means "long-lasting," and "obstructive" means that the ease with which air can flow into and out of the lungs is abnormally reduced.

Is COPD common?

Yes. COPD has been diagnosed in roughly 16 million Americans, and it is estimated that double that number have the condition. It is the fourth leading cause of death in the United States, causing 123,013 deaths in 2001.

What are COPD's worst effects?

A constant, exhausting state of breathlessness in which the victim, to maintain labored breathing, is forced to use the shoulder muscles to try to increase chest movement. In the end, an oxygen mask or mechanical assistance may be needed in order to breathe. COPD causes much distress, suffering, and disability, and takes a heavy economic toll—in 2000 the United States spent $30.4 billion on it.

Is COPD reversible?

No, but treatment can slow down its progression if it is caught early. To find out if treatment is likely to help, the spirometry test can be repeated after giving the patient a bronchodilator, widening the lungs' air passages. If the maximum air that a patient can breath out rises more than 12 percent, this shows a not too serious obstruction and that treatment could well be effective.

DAMAGE TO THE LUNGS FROM COPD

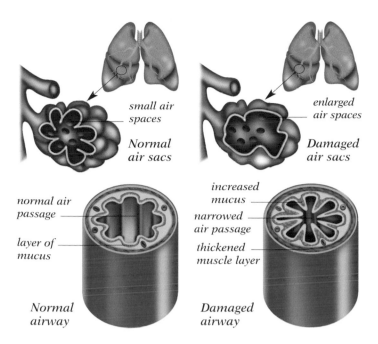

▲ *In COPD, the lungs' air sacs become stretched and the area where oxygen is absorbed is reduced. Also, the air passages are narrowed, owing to the thickened walls and increased mucus.*

infections. The condition usually takes about 10 years of regular smoking to develop, although it can take a shorter time than this.

Symptoms

The symptoms vary with the severity of the obstruction. The first signs of danger are usually a persistent cough—often referred to as "smoker's cough"—and the regular production of sputum. Other symptoms include a feeling of tightness in the chest, breathlessness on minor physical exertion (dyspnea), a high-pitched breathing sound known as wheezing, and awareness of the increased effort required for breathing. The skin, lips, and nails may show a blue tinge—a condition called cyanosis. Another sign is the development of a barrel chest, as the lungs become enlarged and force the diaphragm downward, preventing it from contracting efficiently. The brain's function may also be affected by a combination of not enough oxygen and too much carbon dioxide in the blood, which can cause headaches, insomnia, and impaired mental ability. Extreme coughing fits may occasionally result in hemoptysis (the coughing up of blood), along with the sputum.

In severe cases of COPD pressure on the pulmonary artery increases until the right ventricle of the heart cannot contract efficiently and is thus unable to pump enough blood into the kidneys and legs. This results in swollen feet, ankles, and lower legs (edema). Weight loss may also occur because the huge effort to breathe burns up many calories.

Main methods of diagnosis

If a patient reveals any of the symptoms linked with COPD, then the doctor may decide to carry out pulmonary function tests (PFTs) to confirm a diagnosis. One of the most reliable PFTs is spirometry, which measures the amount of air entering and leaving the lungs.

The patient sits in front of a machine called a spirometer, which is connected to a wide tube, and breathes in to the fullest extent possible before exhaling the entire (maximal) breath into the tube as fast and forcefully as possible. The spirometer accurately measures the volume of air exhaled in 1 second, which is known as the FEV1 (forced expiratory volume in 1 second). When the maximum volume of air that can be expelled from the lungs is measured for a period of 1 second, it provides a useful clinical assessment of the ease with which air can flow through the lungs' airways. The total amount of air that a person can breathe out after taking a maximal breath is called the FVC (forced vital capacity). In a healthy person the FEV1 is about 80 percent of the FVC. In a person with obstructive lung disease FEV1 will be less than 80 percent of FVC.

The patient's lung volumes may also be tested, either by gas dilution or by body plethysmography. In the gas dilution test the patient inhales a gas, such as nitrogen or helium, and the doctor measures the volume in which it is distributed to determine the volume of air that the lungs can hold. In body plethysmography the patient sits in an airtight chamber and inhales and exhales into a tube. A machine called a plethosmograph records changes in pressure, which are used to calculate the volume of air in the lungs. The most important measurements recorded are the residual volume and the TLC (total lung capacity). An increased residual volume shows that air is being trapped, indicating that exhalation is being obstructed. A high TLC shows that the lungs are hyperinflated—a sign of emphysema.

Blood tests, which measure the amount of oxygen and carbon dioxide in the blood, and chest X rays, which reveal lung damage, are also used to identify COPD.

Treatment

First and foremost, the patient must not smoke or be exposed to cigarette smoke. The patient is often given bronchodilators, as well as antibiotics to avoid any infection of the lung secretions. Inhaled corticosteroids are administered, as with those suffering from asthma, to attack the inflammation of the air tube walls. Supplemental oxygen may also be given to the patient to inhale. In some cases, people in the last stage of COPD may have to rely on mechanical assistance to breathe.

Progress of the disease

Clinically, the disease can be divided into three stages. The forced expiratory volume (FEV) is used to measure the progress of COPD within the body. In stage 1 the FEV is greater than or equal to 50 percent of normal lung function. In stage 2 it is 35 to 49 percent, and in stage 3 it is less than 35 percent of predicted normal lung function. Increased resistance to the flow of blood through the lungs causes abnormal strain on the heart, and a form of heart failure called cor pulmonale may develop. The plight of those who reach stage 3 is very distressing. They struggle for breath even when reclining, the shoulders heave and neck muscles strain to maintain the necessary effort for respiration, and the skin is blue with cyanosis. Their condition worsens until even the relief of an oxygen mask will no longer be enough help for them to breathe properly. Ultimately they will die from the disease.

See also: **Antibiotics; Asthma; Blood; Breathing; Bronchitis; Chest; Coughing; Emphysema; Heart disease; Pulmonary disorders; Smoking; Wheezing**

Circulatory system

Questions and Answers

My mother sometimes complains of pins and needles. Is something wrong with her circulation?

The pricking sensation of pins and needles is actually the irritation of a nerve, caused when blood supply is restricted for some reason. This often comes about through lying in an awkward position, but it can also be a sign of circulatory disease that has damaged the blood vessels. If the problem persists, your mother should see a doctor.

I am heavy. My doctor has warned me that my weight is harmful to my circulation. Why is this?

When you are overweight, you carry too much fat. The surplus fat must have a blood supply, so additional and unnecessary blood vessels open up. Obesity is also associated with the serious arterial disease atherosclerosis, which can narrow arteries. This causes further problems: to keep the blood flowing around the system, the heart has to do extra work, which may strain it. A heavy body also requires more effort to move around, and this, too, could strain the heart. To avoid these risks, shed the extra pounds.

My teenage daughter keeps on fainting, but she looks completely healthy. Do you think she might have problems with her circulation?

The most usual cause of fainting is a temporary fall in the volume of blood reaching the brain. This is a common problem in adolescents, particularly girls. It is often caused by emotional disturbance, which can make the arteries widen, lowering the blood pressure and preventing blood from being pumped up to the brain. Girls usually grow out of this sort of fainting, but if the fainting spells increase or your daughter is worried that she may be ill, she should see her doctor promptly.

Blood pumped by the heart is continuously circulating around the body. Its journey has several essential purposes—among them, to supply the body's cells with food and oxygen and to clear them of waste products.

The circulatory system is a closed network of blood vessels—tubes that carry blood around the body. At its center is the heart, a muscular pump that keeps the blood constantly moving on its journey.

Arteries and arterioles

Blood begins its journey around the circulatory system by leaving the left side of the heart through the large artery known as the aorta. At this stage blood is rich in oxygen, in food broken down into the microscopically small components called molecules, and in vital substances such as hormones.

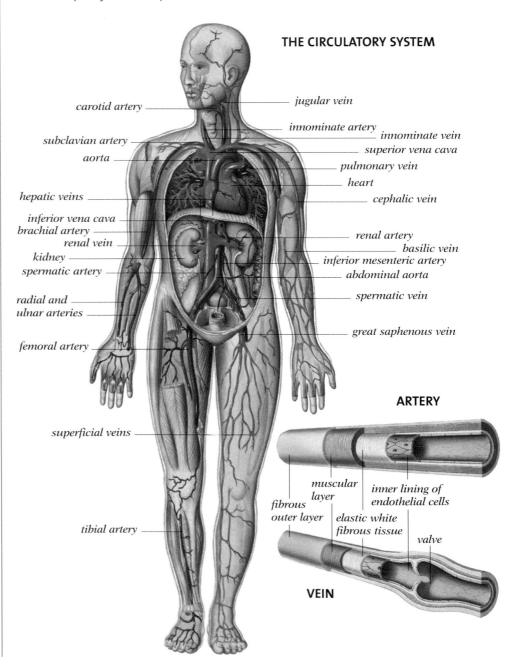

THE CIRCULATORY SYSTEM

carotid artery
jugular vein
innominate artery
innominate vein
subclavian artery
superior vena cava
aorta
pulmonary vein
heart
hepatic veins
cephalic vein
inferior vena cava
brachial artery
renal artery
renal vein
basilic vein
kidney
inferior mesenteric artery
spermatic artery
abdominal aorta
spermatic vein
radial and
ulnar arteries
great saphenous vein
femoral artery
superficial veins
ARTERY
muscular
layer
inner lining of
endothelial cells
fibrous
outer layer
elastic white
fibrous tissue
valve
tibial artery
VEIN

DISTRIBUTION OF BLOOD IN THE BODY

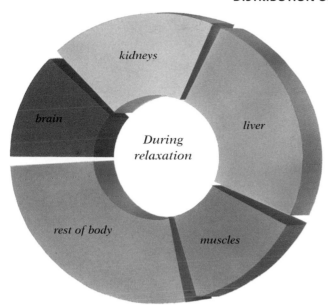
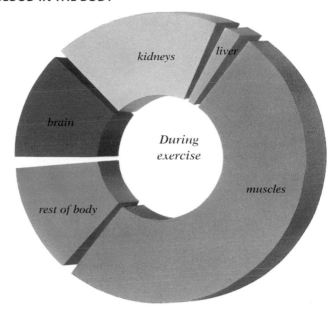

▲ *Blood circulation throughout the body is automatically regulated according to certain activities, so that it is always in the places where it is most needed.*

In the early part of its journey, blood flows through fairly large tubes called arteries. It then passes into smaller ones known as arterioles, which lead to every organ and tissue in the body, including the heart. From here, it enters a vast network of tiny vessels called capillaries, where oxygen and vital molecules are exchanged for waste products.

The veins

Blood then leaves the capillaries and flows into the small veins, or venules, where it starts the journey back to the heart. All the veins from the various parts of the body eventually merge into two large blood vessels: the superior vena cava and the inferior vena cava. The first collects blood from the head, arms, and neck, and the second receives blood from the lower part of the body. Both veins deliver blood to the right side of the heart. From here it is pumped into the pulmonary artery (the only artery to carry blood with no oxygen), which takes the blood to the lungs, where oxygen from air breathed in is absorbed into it, and the waste product, carbon dioxide, is released and breathed out.

The journey's final stage is for the now oxygen-rich blood to flow through the pulmonary vein (the only vein to carry oxygenated blood) into the left side of the heart, where it starts its circuit once again.

Distribution

Blood is not spread evenly throughout the system. At any given time there is about 11 percent in the arteries, 12 percent in the lungs, 61 percent in veins and venules, 7 percent in arterioles and capillaries, and 9 percent in the heart. Blood also flows at different rates. It spurts from the heart and through the aorta at 13 inches (33 cm) per second, slows down to 0.1 inches (0.25 cm) per second when reaching the capillaries, then flows back through the veins to gradually reach 8 inches (20 cm) per second when it gets to the heart.

Pulse and blood pressure

One of the main guides a doctor has to the condition of a patient's circulation is the pulse, for it is a mirror of the heartbeat. Arteries have elastic walls that expand every time the heart pumps a wave of blood through them. It is possible to feel this happening if an artery near the body's surface is found, such as at the wrist, and pressed against a bone.

The normal pulse rate is between 60 and 80 beats a minute but varies widely. Thus a doctor taking a pulse is not only counting the beats but feeling for changes in their strength and regularity.

Blood pressure is different from pulse rate—it is a measurement of the force with which the heart pumps blood into the arteries. A blood pressure measurement is often taken on the upper arm because here a suitable artery is in a situation in which it can be readily compressed. The instrument for measuring blood pressure consequently works on the principle that if the flow of blood through the artery is temporarily closed (by inflating a special encircling bag around the arm), the sound made by the initial movement of blood through the compressed artery, as the pressure is gradually released, indicates the point at which the pressure in the artery and in the compression bag are the same. A gauge attached to the bag indicates the pressure.

If the blood pressure is higher than normal, the heart is probably having to work harder to push the blood through the system, perhaps indicating a disease in the circulatory system, such as narrowing of the arteries (see Blood Pressure). The smaller the opening in a blood vessel, the harder the heart has to work to pump the blood through it. If the heart works too hard for a long period of time, its life may be shortened, and this is why doctors constantly look out for high blood pressure.

Further controls

The width of blood vessels also controls circulation. Changes in width are caused by two means: hormones and nerves. If blood pressure drops, the kidneys emit a hormone called angiotensin, which causes the arteries to narrow and the blood pressure to return to normal rate.

See also: **Arteries and artery disease; Blood; Body structure; Brain; Capillaries; Coronary arteries and thrombosis; Heart; Hormones; Kidneys and kidney diseases; Lung and lung diseases; Oxygen; Pulmonary disorders; Pulse; Veins**

Circumcision

Questions and Answers

If our baby is a boy, my husband wants him to be circumcised. Will this be painful?

On a young baby the area of foreskin is so minute that the infant will hardly notice. A dressing is applied immediately, so there should be no infection.

My boyfriend is circumcised and insists that it makes him a better lover. Is this true?

There is no scientific evidence to show that a man who has been circumcised has a firmer erection or a better technique than an uncircumcised man.

I heard that a woman married to a circumcised man is less likely to get cervical cancer. Is this true?

This belief has been held for a long time, many people arguing that Jewish women have a much lower risk of this kind of cancer because their husbands are circumcised. But two studies, one American and one British, failed to show any difference in the incidence of cancer of the cervix between wives of circumcised men and wives of uncircumcised men.

What is female circumcision?

In girls, the clitoris—a small organ situated in front of the urethra—also has a hood like the male penis, but there are no reasons for its removal. "Female circumcision" is a religious or cultural practice common in some countries, although it is considered barbaric in the West. It may involve the removal of the clitoris or the sewing together of the vaginal lips, or both. It makes intercourse very painful for women, and a woman has to be "opened up" for childbirth and resewn afterward, causing terrible pain and a high risk of infection.

Circumcision, the cutting away of the foreskin of the penis, is practiced the world over, mainly for religious reasons. Although a safe procedure, the operation is increasingly carried out only for medical reasons in the West.

Boys are born with a sheath or hood covering the glans, or tip, of the penis. This is the foreskin, or prepuce, which extends from the skin of the penis. It reaches forward over the glans, then turns back onto the penis itself. In the nonerect penis, the foreskin has to be pulled back to expose the glans. Circumcision refers to a cutting away of the foreskin so that the glans is permanently exposed. In a baby it is a quick and almost painless procedure. In older children and adults an anesthetic is needed during the operation.

Religious reasons
Circumcision may be carried out for religious reasons or because of health or medical problems. Worldwide, the largest religious group practicing circumcision is Muslims. Circumcision is also practiced by Jews, preferably when a baby is between two and 10 days old. Orthodox Jews have their sons circumcised during religious ceremonies, when the boys are eight days old.

Circumcision and health
In the United States circumcision is performed principally as a measure to aid hygiene, because washing beneath the foreskin can be overlooked. However, the American Academy of Pediatrics states that routine circumcision is unnecessary. Nowadays, in the United Kingdom and many other countries, circumcisions are performed mainly for medical reasons.

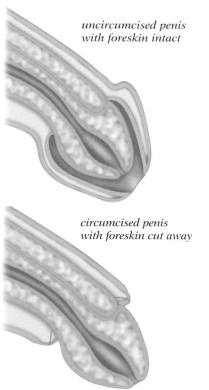

uncircumcised penis with foreskin intact

circumcised penis with foreskin cut away

▲ *In an uncircumcised male, the foreskin of the nonerect penis covers the glans, or tip. Circumcision exposes the glans.*

The most common medical reason for circumcision is in the case of phimosis, or the inability to pull back the foreskin. Phimosis is more likely after inflammation of the glans and foreskin, a condition called balanitis. Circumcision in this case is best carried out at age three to five years, although the condition may arise later in childhood or in adulthood.

Paraphimosis is a condition in which a pulled-back foreskin cannot be brought forward over the glans. This may cause painful swelling of the penis tip. The patient may need to go to the hospital for a slit of the upper part of the foreskin, carried out under an anesthetic.

Aftercare
Removal of the foreskin leaves a raw area on the penis that requires daily care. In a baby, irritation from a wet diaper or the presence of infection in the urine means there is a risk that a small ulcer will form at the tip of the penis. The baby requires frequent diaper changes and more frequent bathing during the healing period. Local dressing of the sore area of the penis is usually advised by the doctor (see Sores). However, it is not necessary to dress the wound while it heals. Generally, the risk of infection is slight.

See also: Anesthetics; Erection and ejaculation; Genital mutilation; Healing; Infection and infectious diseases; Penis and disorders; Ulcers

Cirrhosis

Questions and Answers

How much can I drink before I develop cirrhosis of the liver? Does it matter what alcohol I drink?

French experts estimate that the consumption of about 1½ oz. (40 g) of pure alcohol a day for up to 10 years will cause cirrhosis in most people. This is the equivalent of drinking 10 beers or 10 whiskeys every day for that period. What matters is the total quantity of alcohol consumed: the choice of drink makes no difference.

I have been a heavy drinker for some time. How do I know whether my liver is damaged?

There are usually no symptoms in mild cirrhosis, and simple blood tests will not indicate how much permanent damage has been done. The only sure way of making a diagnosis is to have a small piece of the liver examined under a microscope. This may not be necessary. Talk to your doctor about your drinking and cut down. Or better, stop altogether.

My father has been told that his heavy drinking has affected his liver. Is there any chance that it may recover?

This depends very much on the severity of the damage. Liver cells do possess a tremendous capacity to repair damage, but it is unlikely that a cirrhotic liver will be able to replace all the lost tissue. Once the cirrhotic process takes hold, the disease is irreversible.

I had cirrhosis over a year ago. Can I start to drink again?

No, not if you truly have cirrhosis; the disease is not reversible. However, if you had a bout of jaundice, due to hepatitis, without permanent damage, you may resume drinking if your doctor says there is no serious risk.

Although cirrhosis of the liver can develop after a bout of infectious hepatitis, the disease mostly affects heavy drinkers. If left untreated, this condition can result in permanent liver damage and death.

Cirrhosis is a liver disease characterized by a progressive destruction of liver cells (hepatocytes). These are then replaced with fibrous tissue, which gradually leads to hardening and reduced effectiveness of the organ. Clumps of small nodules give the cirrhotic liver a knobbly appearance.

Causes

The most common cause of cirrhosis is alcoholism. The quantity of alcohol needed to damage the liver varies with each individual, but drinking for 10 years at a rate of 10 cans of beer (or 10 single shots of whiskey) each day will probably cause cirrhosis. Viral hepatitis can also lead to cirrhosis. The virus responsible may be transmitted in blood from hypodermic needles or blood transfusions, and in contaminated drinking water. Type A hepatitis rarely causes cirrhosis.

Symptoms and dangers

In mild cirrhosis there are usually no symptoms. The onset of the disease is gradual, and many of the symptoms are a result of toxic chemicals accumulating in the body, and of internal bleeding, due to lack of the necessary clotting factors in the blood. As the condition progresses, brain function is impaired, and bile accumulates in the skin, causing severe itching, followed by jaundice and the contraction of the liver. The abdomen swells, and fine red lines, caused by small veins, appear on the skin.

In men, the testicles may shrink and the breasts may begin to grow, because the liver is no longer able to cope with the small amounts of female hormone that are normally present in the body.

In the most severe cases of cirrhosis, death can result, either from an irreversible coma or from bleeding. This latter is caused by the rupturing of the enlarged veins around the esophagus (gullet). Cirrhosis is also a major cause of cancer of the liver.

Treatment and outlook

When cirrhosis is brought on by alcohol abuse, the treatment is abstinence (see Alcoholism). Protection against type B viral hepatitis can be given by vaccination or, in an emergency, by an injection of gamma globulin, which is rich in antibodies against the virus. However, once the cirrhotic process is fully established, there is no effective treatment except a liver transplant. The liver cells possess a great capacity to repair damage, but ultimately cell destruction outstrips cell replacement. Once the cirrhotic process is past this point, death usually follows within 10 years.

> *See also:* Bile; Blood transfusion; Cancer; Cells and chromosomes; Esophagus; Hepatitis; Hormones; Immunization; Infection and infectious diseases; Jaundice; Liver and liver diseases; Veins

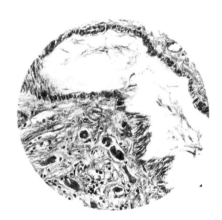

▲ *A microscopic section of liver tissue affected by cirrhosis.*

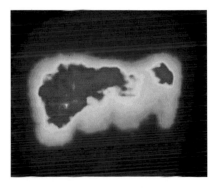

▲ *An image of a cirrhotic liver taken using radioactive isotopes.*

Cleft palate

Questions and Answers

Will my daughter's cleft palate affect her speech?

Not if surgery is performed early enough to repair the damage. After her operation, your daughter's progress will be checked regularly; if she is not developing normal speech, she will receive speech therapy. The chances of her having normal or nearly normal speech by the time she goes to school are very good.

My baby has a cleft palate. Does this mean I can't breast-feed him?

Your baby may find it difficult to breast-feed at first, but he should be able to manage with some practice. If problems persist, try spoon-feeding. It may also help to lay your baby on his stomach when he is feeding, because this reduces the chance that milk will go down the air passage.

My first child had a cleft lip. Does this mean my next child will have the same defect? Does the fact that I am 38 make it more likely?

If neither you nor your partner had a cleft lip, then the chance that your next child will have one is slim. If, however, either of you had a cleft and your child had the same type of cleft, there is a 15 percent risk that your next child will inherit it. There is no evidence to suggest that a mother's age causes any type of cleft.

What kind of problems should I expect my baby, who has a cleft palate, to have?

Sometimes a child with a cleft palate also exhibits mental retardation, deafness, or both in addition to poor health. But provided he or she does not have other problems, once the palate has been repaired, your child should develop normally.

One in every 2,500 babies is born with a cleft palate, a cleft lip, or both these conditions. Surgery can improve appearance, while speech therapy helps the child overcome any communication problems.

The palate is the roof of the mouth. The front part is hard and is called the hard palate; the back part is soft and is called the soft palate. Most of the hard palate is formed as part of the upper jawbone, whereas the soft palate is made of muscle (see Palate). The soft palate is lifted up to close the back of the nose when a person swallows, and it is lowered to let air escape through the nose to produce the sounds "n," "m," and "ng."

Causes and symptoms

The early embryo is a tubelike structure. Early in fetal life the face develops when a finger of tissue grows in from either side to fuse with a central nasal process growing down from above. These processes can fail to fuse properly at various points, causing a gap which may involve the upper lip, the palate, or both. Clefts run in families, with relatives often showing the same type of cleft. Cleft lip is more common in boys and cleft palate in girls.

Symptoms

Clefts are divided into types, depending on where they occur—in the lip only, in the ridge behind the teeth (alveolar), or in the palate. All three types can occur together. However, because the palate joins in the front part, and then closes forward toward the lip and back to the soft palate and uvula (the flap of tissue that helps to prevent food from entering the air passages during swallowing), clefts are more common in the lip and uvula than in the front part of the palate.

The seriousness of the cleft can vary—from a groove in the lip or uvula to a complete separation of the two halves of the palate and lip. Clefts can be one-sided or two-sided. The latter occur in alveolar clefts and lip clefts, with a cleft on either side of the two front teeth.

At birth these clefts are clearly visible, unlike a submucous cleft, where the muscles of the palate have not joined but the skin covering the palate has. This condition may cause speech problems.

Outlook

Because nearly all clefts are repaired early in infancy, it is extremely rare for an adult to be left with an obvious deformity or poor speech. After surgery and dental work, speech will usually develop normally. When there are special difficulties and the child has not achieved normal or nearly normal speech by the age of four or five, therapy may be required.

> See also: **Birth defects; Bones; Fetus; Heredity; Mouth; Muscles; Nose; Speech; Speech therapy; Teeth and teething**

NORMAL PALATE

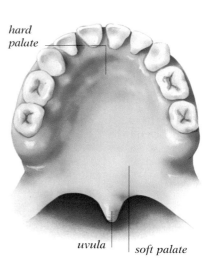

hard palate

uvula · soft palate

CLEFT PALATE

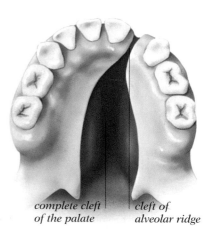

complete cleft of the palate · cleft of alveolar ridge

▲ *Unlike a normal palate (top), a cleft palate has a separation between the two sides (above).*

Cloning

The cloning revolution really started when Scottish scientists at the Roslin Institute created the sheep clone Dolly in 1996. Was Dolly the first animal to be artificially cloned?

No. Embryo cloning of mice, which produced identical mouse clones, had been going on since the late 1970s. Similar cloning of larger animals had been in progress since the late 1980s.

So why all the fuss about Dolly?

Embryo clones are like identical twins. In Dolly's case, however, a clone of an adult animal was made. This method, called nuclear transfer, is an entirely different process with much wider implications. The reason for public interest in Dolly was that it raised the controversial possibility of producing human clones.

How many animals have now been cloned?

Several thousands. By the end of 2000 at least 5,000 clones of mammals had been produced, including mice, sheep, pigs, goats, cows, monkeys, and rats.

Isn't animal cloning immoral?

This is a difficult question. If you believe that an activity is justified by substantial human benefits, then the answer is no. Animal cloning has many benefits. It can provide an unlimited supply of transgenic animals and their organs for use in human transplantation. It can produce stem cells (cells that can be developed into any kind of body cell) that have the potential to cure many human diseases for which there is no current remedy, and it can increase our understanding of genetics, which has already led to benefits for humankind.

Although natural cloning of simple organisms has occured for millions of years, it has only recently become possible to clone large and complex animals, including humans, artificially.

Human cloning is the production of genetically identical humans. An example of cloning is the case of identical twins. After a human egg cell (ovum) has been fertilized it begins to divide. Sometimes, after the first division, the two resulting cells, instead of sticking together, separate to form two individual cells. Each of these then continues to divide separately from the other so that two full normal individuals are produced. Because these twins have exactly the same DNA, they are physically identical and are called clones. This process is called cloning by twinning, or embryo cloning. It is one of the ways in which artificial clones can be made.

Features of clones

Clones have identical DNA and share all the physical features that are brought about by the genes in the DNA. The study of identical twins has shown that clones' identity is not limited to purely physical characteristics; human clones also tend to think alike and to have similar artistic tastes. These studies have been valuable in showing which features of an individual are not of genetic origin but are the result of environmental influences. The same applies to all clones. The adult clone is a result of the way all the experiences of the individual modify the state of the genetically determined being.

How cloning is done

Embryo cloning duplicates the natural process that produces identical twins. The process must be done before the cells of the embryo differentiate—while they are, in effect, still stem cells. After fertilization, the early cell mass is divided into pieces that can each form a complete and normal individual. Using a process known as the polymerase chain reaction (PCR), machines can

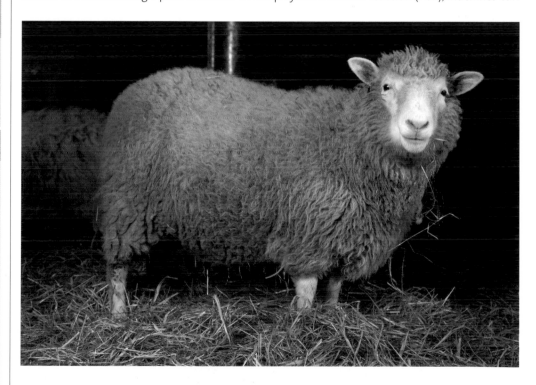

▲ *The famous sheep Dolly, 1996–2003, was the first clone of an adult mammal ever produced. The method used for this process is called nuclear cell transfer.*

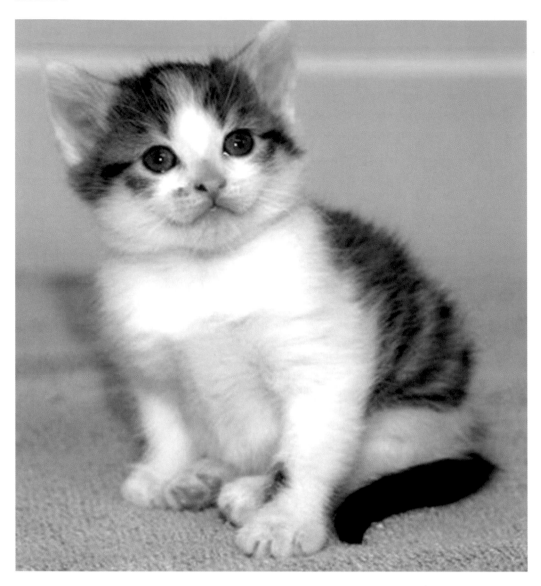

◀ *CC is the first domestic cat ever to be cloned. She was born on December 22, 2001, in Texas.*

the cutting. Its DNA is the same. Many single-celled species, such as bacteria and fungi, reproduce by cloning. Their DNA duplicates itself and splits off, and the new genome forms the DNA of the new individual. Since genes were first isolated as lengths of DNA, most of them have been cloned.

Purpose of cloning research

Cloning research has already added greatly to doctors' knowledge of human reproduction, and it has the potential to make the treatment of infertility much more effective and successful. In the future, the transmission of severe genetic defects may be prevented by inserting specific genes into cells that produce sperm or eggs, or into early embryos. Potentially, twins could even be produced to order (see Genetics).

With regard to cell replication, a greater understanding of biochemical reactions may result in new and better forms of contraception. Cloning may also provide a backup of early embryos that could be frozen and kept indefinitely for possible future use, or it may provide a long-term source of stem cells that could be used by the donor or by anyone else. Cloned animals could be genetically engineered to produce valuable drugs and surgically useful organs and tissues.

produce millions of gene clones. These machines are in use all over the world and are indispensable in medical research.

Another cloning method

Cloning of an adult mammal requires a totally different process, called nuclear cell transfer. A healthy egg (ovum) is a single cell containing the DNA contribution from the mother. The DNA is removed and the whole nucleus of a cell is taken from the part of the body of the individual to be cloned; this is then inserted into the ovum. The ovum now contains the complete DNA genome of the donor. Various techniques, such as electrical pulsation, are used to cause the ovum to start dividing as if it were a normal fertilized egg. Once division has started, the ovum is implanted in the uterus of a female of the same species as the donor. This is a much simplified way of describing a very complicated process. If all goes well and the pregnancy comes to term, the baby will be a clone of the donor individual.

Cloning in nature

Gardeners have been cloning for hundreds of years. When they take a cutting from a plant and persuade it to grow, they are producing a new individual that is a clone of the plant from which they took

Potential benefits and problems of cloning

There has been much speculation about the ways human cloning could benefit mankind. These are: the use of stem cells to produce organs or tissues to repair or to replace damaged ones; help for infertile couples who want to have children; the production of bone, fat, and tissues for plastic and cosmetic surgery; and cloning to prevent diseases and syndromes caused by defective genes or recessive genetic disorders. However, there are many problems to be overcome before the full potential of cloning can truly be realized. Every major new development in this field runs the risk of abuse, and there are also ethical and possibly moral dangers inherent in the process of cloning. What is becoming apparent is that the possibility of cloning humans is no longer science fiction.

> *See also:* **Bacteria; Cells and chromosomes; Conception; Cosmetic surgery; Genetic diseases and disorders; Genetic engineering; Infertility; In vitro fertilization**

Clubfoot

Questions and Answers

My baby was born with a clubfoot, which has now been corrected. Is my next child likely to have the same condition?

No. This is just another old wives' tale. Ask your doctor about genetic counseling, which is provided for parents worried about these risks.

I had a bad fright while I was pregnant. Could this be the reason my son has a clubfoot? Or was it something to do with my diet?

It is extremely unlikely that a bad fright caused the problem. There is also nothing to suggest that nutritional deficiencies during pregnancy play a part. Doctors think the deformity is due to a halt in the foot's development.

I have heard that if a child has a clubfoot, his or her foot can be put in a plaster cast to set it into the correct position. Is this true?

Doctors sometimes use this method, but it is only part of the treatment for the condition. Repeated manipulation is more important to coax the foot into the correct position. Casts and splints may then be used to maintain the position if necessary.

If a child has a clubfoot, is he or she likely to have other physical or mental disabilities?

The answer depends on whether this is an isolated deformity—as is usually the case. A few cases of clubfoot are linked with other disorders, such as congenital dislocation of the hip, or may arise through conditions such as cerebral palsy or spina bifida (a defect in the spinal wall). Where clubfoot occurs by itself, there is no reason to fear that the child will be mentally retarded or affected in any other way.

A small number of babies are born with a clubfoot. Why this condition occurs is not fully understood, but it can be corrected—sometimes very easily—if treated early enough.

The term "clubfoot" (medically, congenital talipes) is applied to a deformity, present at birth, in which the bones in the ankle are incorrectly placed. When this happens, the sole of the foot faces inward and the toes point down. The cause of clubfoot is not known. It is likely that several factors play a part—for example, there may be some hereditary influence. Early theories suggested that clubfoot might result from the fetus's lying in an abnormal position, or that it might be due to pressure on the fetus because of lack of uterine fluid. However, a deficiency of fluid often occurs without any resulting deformity, and it is known that the fetus constantly moves its limbs while in the womb.

A halt in the development of the feet may be part of the explanation—there is a stage in the normal growth of the feet when they do appear to be clubbed. However, there is no known reason why this arrest might occur.

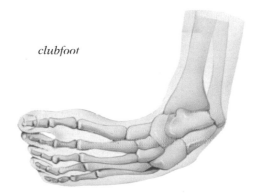

normal foot

clubfoot

▲ *In a clubfoot, the bones in the ankle are in the wrong position, causing the ankle to twist. Usually, the foot is bent downward, and the sole faces inward.*

Symptoms

In the typical clubfoot, the foot is bent downward and the ankle twisted, so that the sole faces inward. In a few instances a doctor or physical therapist can manipulate the foot into the normal position. Such cases usually recover in a few weeks with a minimum of help. However, in most cases the condition cannot be fully corrected so easily and will need more prolonged treatment. Occasionally the foot is deformed in the other direction—it is bent upward and the sole faces outward. Another type of deformity affects the front part of the foot only. It is important for a doctor to distinguish these problems as soon after birth as possible. Without attention, the deformity may progress, and the child will develop an abnormal gait (see Splints).

Treatment

The earlier treatment starts the better. In the first few weeks of life the deformity may respond to fairly simple measures. Repeated gentle stretching of the foot will encourage it into the correct position, while bandaging between stretches will help keep it there. Doctors sometimes use splints and plaster of paris to achieve a good position. When the child starts to walk, he or she may need special shoes to maintain the best foot position. When simple measures fail to correct the condition, surgery may be needed to prevent the deformity from becoming permanent. This is required in around 50 percent of cases, but an operation is almost always successful.

See also: Birth; Birth defects; Bones; Congenital disorders; Feet; Growth; Heredity; Hip; Orthopedics; Pediatric medicine; Surgery

Cocaine and crack

Cocaine and crack are dangerous drugs that are in general use among drug abusers. Crack, in particular, has become increasingly common in recent years, and causes great social and criminal problems.

Cocaine, once exclusive to the working people of the Andes of South America, has become the most widely abused dangerous drug in the Western world. The use of its purified form—crack—is now commonplace. Cocaine is a natural alkaloid derived from the leaves of *Erythroxylon coca* and *E. truxiuense*, small shrublike trees indigenous to Columbia, Peru, and Bolivia. For centuries the hard-working natives of these countries have chewed the leaves of the coca plant to increase their endurance, relieve their hunger, improve their strength, and promote a sense of well-being. Cocaine was rarely used as a recreational drug until the late 1960s, when the cost of amphetamines became prohibitive as a result of federal restrictions on its illegal distribution. By the late 1980s, almost 20 percent of young adults had used cocaine at least once, and 5 percent were using it regularly. Usage has become far more widespread.

The effects of the drug

Cocaine acts upon the neurotransmitter dopamine, which stimulates the brain. Cocaine blocks the re-uptake of dopamine into the nerve endings in the brain. This uptake normally reduces the ability of dopamine to stimulate the brain, so cocaine, by blocking its re-uptake, increases stimulation. The effects are similar to those of amphetamines, but less persistent.

Cocaine and Freud

Cocaine was largely unknown to Western medicine until the Austrian psychiatrist Sigmund Freud became interested in it. In 1883 he tried the drug to see if he could relieve his habitual tiredness, depression, and stomach cramps. To his delight, all his symptoms disappeared. The results impressed him so much that he began to prescribe cocaine to friends, colleagues, patients with heart disease, and those with "nervous exhaustion" following morphine withdrawal. The only effect was to substitute cocaine addiction for morphine addiction. Undaunted, Freud continued his research. He concluded that the greatest value of the drug was in temporarily strengthening the body. He also recommended it to relieve indigestion and

▼ *Here free-based cocaine is put in a pipe and lit before being smoked.*

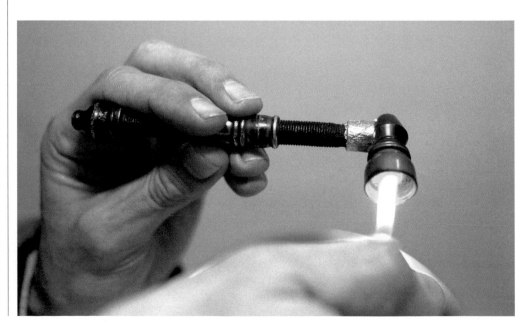

Questions and Answers

Can cocaine and crack affect the ability to drive safely?

Yes. Research in Memphis has shown that a high percentage of males arrested for reckless driving had substantial levels of cocaine in their bloodstreams. Most were found to be intoxicated, too, although, for the purposes of the study, all cases of alcoholic intoxication were excluded. The figures showed a high level of cocaine usage.

Do police tests for alcoholic intoxication reveal cocaine use?

No, but this is a growing danger to the public and a concern to medical and legal authorities.

Why do the media always connect cocaine with crime?

Cocaine and crack are illegal drugs, sold by criminals. The trade is so lucrative that they will go to any lengths, including murder, to promote it. Cocaine and crack are expensive, and many users cannot legally find the money for their habit, so they may resort to burglary, mugging, prostitution, or extortion to get it.

Why do cocaine users laugh when I suggest that it is dangerous?

Recreational users of moderate doses of cocaine rarely suffer more than minor side effects, and these may seem unimportant to them. Some users, however, find that they cannot continue on small doses, may resort to crack, and may increase the amount taken. They are likely to damage themselves in one way or another.

Where did crack get its name?

When crack is heated for smoking, it makes a crackling sound.

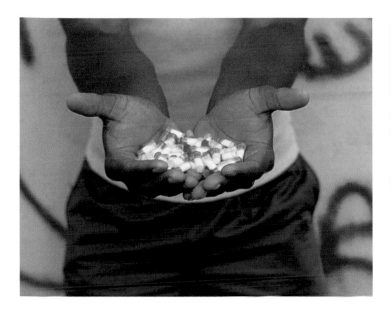

▲ *The consequences of crack usage are serious: it is an illegal drug with serious medical problems, including addiction.*

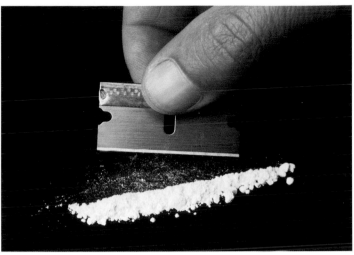

▲ *Cocaine hydrochloride is chopped up before being snorted.*

to treat anemia, asthma, and alcohol and morphine addiction. He was convinced that the drug was an aphrodisiac. Having noticed the numbing effect of the drug on the mouth, Freud recognized its possible value as a local anesthetic, but because he left the promotion of this application to a colleague, he was denied credit for what proved the only valid medical use of the drug (see Anesthetics). Ironically, the other uses he suggested came to be seen by himself and others as undesirable and misguided.

After about 1886 Freud no longer took cocaine or recommended it as a general stimulant. The drug, however, soon became widely popular as a mental stimulant and promoter of a "high." It is prepared by mashing coca leaves, dissolving out the drug, and preparing the hydrochloride salt. Illegally imported in that form, it is then cut with inert materials to increase its bulk and street value.

Crack and addiction

Crack is a highly purified and powerful form of cocaine extracted from the cruder product with alkaline water or ether. It is volatile when heated and is readily absorbed through the lungs—a high results, with a short period of intense pleasure. This feeling is strongest on the first use and is not experienced to the same intensity again. The intensity of the sensation is matched by its danger, and the incidence of toxic effects is much higher than with the weaker preparation. Crack quickly leads to dependence in some users, and there is no way of knowing in advance who will become addicted and who will not.

Some people seem to have little difficulty in keeping usage under control, but approximately 15 percent of users take larger and larger doses until they are as dependent on the drug as heroin addicts. Laboratory animals, given the choice of injecting themselves with cocaine or taking food, prefer the cocaine and continue to inject it until they are exhausted or dead.

The likelihood of severe addiction depends on how the drug is taken. People who are smoking crack (freebasing) or injecting it (shooting) are much more likely to become addicted than those who are only snorting the drug. In freebasing, up to 80 percent of the dose can get to the brain in about 10 seconds. As with any other major drug, addiction may lead to serious medical, social, financial, and legal consequences.

Medical effects

Cocaine increases the heart rate and narrows the blood vessels, raising the blood pressure. It initially widens the air passages in the lungs and shrinks the lining of the nose, making breathing easier. After use, however, there is a rebound stuffiness of the nose and a tendency to resort to the drug to relieve it. The effects of the high dopamine levels on the brain are identical to those of amphetamine. Euphoria, increased awareness, and mental stimulation are strong, and there is a decreased sense of fatigue. Motor activity is increased but coordination is reduced.

Many people imagine that cocaine and crack are harmless. Medical evidence shows, however, that they are often extremely dangerous, and this is especially true of crack. The most common physical effects include epileptic-type fits, loss of consciousness, running and bleeding nose, sore throat, sinusitis, pain in the chest, coughing blood, pneumonia, severe itching ("cocaine bug"), irregularity of the heart, loss of appetite, and stomach upset.

Some of the chest and throat problems are probably caused by the high temperature of the inhaled cocaine fumes. The nose and sinus disorders are due to the constricting effect of cocaine on the blood vessels in the nose lining. This is sometimes severe enough to destroy part of the partition between the two halves of the nose (the columella), leaving a perforation (see Nose). With increasing doses, coordination becomes ever more affected, and tremors and then seizures occur. Eventually the respiratory centers in the brain stem are blocked and death follows from respiratory failure.

Crack can lead to a short-lived, acute form of mental illness called cocaine psychosis. The symptoms include severe depression, agitation, delusions, persecution fantasies, hallucinations, violent behavior, and suicidal intentions. People with cocaine psychosis often have lucid intervals when they appear normal and deny using the drug. This usually follows long binges or high doses of the drug.

See also: Amphetamines; Drug abuse; Drug counseling

381

Cold sores

Questions and Answers

Whenever I get anxious, I feel a prickling sensation in my lower lip and a cold sore comes up. Is there any connection between cold sores and stress and anxiety?

Possibly, but stress itself will not create a cold sore unless your body has learned to use such situations as a trigger. Cold sores are more likely to occur when you are run-down. This fact could account for the feeling of not being able to cope that accompanies anxiety in many people.

I always seem to get a cold sore before a special occasion, when I want to look my best. How can I stop this from happening?

At the first indication of the start of a cold sore, apply aciclovir repeatedly in the form of Zovirax cream. This may prevent a sore from developing. Even if it does not, it is likely to limit the severity.

Do cold sores run in families?

This has not been proved, but the inability to develop sufficient immunity to the virus that causes cold sores may be hereditary.

My mother suffers from cold sores. She insists on kissing my baby whenever she visits, whether she has them or not. Can cold sores be passed on in this way?

Yes, but your mother may do worse than that. If your baby suffers from eczema or has an eczematous tendency, it could even prove fatal. Kaposi's varicellum eruption, a potentially fatal skin disorder, can be caused in this way. No one with an active cold sore should go near a young child who suffers from eczema. Yet most children have come into contact with the cold sore virus by the time they are five and have developed their own immunity to it.

A cold sore is an unsightly nuisance but not a serious health hazard. Many people develop a natural immunity to cold sores, and symptoms can be alleviated in those who are affected.

The term "cold sore" describes a group of blisters that form around the mouth and inside the nose, usually toward the end of a cold—thus their name. The sores can be irritating, unsightly, and very uncomfortable, but they are not dangerous. They are produced by a virus called herpes simplex. Most people have been exposed to the virus by the time they are five years old and build up a natural immunity so that they never produce cold sores. Yet for the minority who suffer from cold sores, they are a real nuisance.

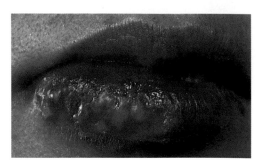

▲ *The typical cold sore is a cluster of tiny blisters that feel itchy and hot, then painful.*

The herpes simplex virus is related to the herpes virus that attacks the genital area. The latter is a sexually transmitted disease, and an immunity to the cold sore virus does not mean that one is immune to genital herpes.

Causes

Once the herpes virus has infected the skin, it remains hidden there, lying dormant between attacks. The body produces a partial immunity that controls the virus for most of the time, until a trigger causes it to flare up. This trigger can be a cold, a bout of flu, a chest infection, or a sore throat. Exposure to sunlight or to harsh winds can also act as a trigger. Some women have a tendency to develop cold sores a few days before or during their menstrual period.

Symptoms

People who have recurring cold sores learn to tell when one is about to begin: there is a sudden, itchy tingling in the skin of the affected area, which can start up to two days before the cold sore erupts. An inflamed cluster of tiny blisters then develops. The blisters fill up with a yellowish-white fluid and feel itchy and hot, a sensation that is followed by tenderness and some pain. Occasionally the inflamed blisters may burst within two to four days of appearing, but in all cases they start to heal by drying up. The sore should be left alone while a crust forms; this will eventually fall off.

Dangers

There is little danger that the skin tissue will scar, except in severe cases. However, it is important to touch the sores as little as possible, as touching may cause them to spread. The protective crust should never be scratched or picked before the sore is fully healed and dried out. If it comes off, the sore could become reinfected, and the healing process would be prolonged unnecessarily.

Treatment

In the early stages before the sore has erupted, while the skin is itching and tingling, the antiviral drug aciclovir, in the form of a cream (trade name Zovirax), may be applied to the affected area to stop the sore from developing further. Zovirax cream is available from pharmacists without a prescription. Applying ice cubes to the tingling area at this stage can also help. Once the blisters appear, nothing will stop them from running their course. There are preparations on the market to relieve the itchiness and pain, but they will not shorten the healing period.

Most cold sores heal naturally within two weeks or so—the process will take no more than three weeks at the most.

See also: Blisters; Herpes; Menstruation; Scars; Sores; Viruses

Colon and colitis

Questions and Answers

I have chronic colitis. Is there a chance my children will catch it?

No. Although the cause of chronic colitis is uncertain—it may be a bacterial infection or a result of psychological disturbance—it is not at all contagious.

If I have chronic colitis, am I likely to get bowel cancer in later life?

It is highly unlikely. Modern drug treatment with salazopyrin is very effective and will usually control the symptoms. If the disease is severe, the colon, or a portion of it, can be removed. Only 5 to 10 percent of those patients who have chronic colitis for 10 years or more develop colonic cancer.

I sometimes have severe diarrhea after I eat certain foods. How can I tell if this is colitis or not?

If you are sure that you are not merely suffering from a stomach upset, and that specific foods trigger diarrhea, you may be having an allergic reaction and be suffering from acute colitis. See your doctor. If the diarrhea is constant, possibly containing mucus, pus, and blood, and you are anemic and dehydrated, you should be examined by your doctor for chronic colitis. The lining of the colon is examined by a colonoscope: the appearance will resemble red velvet and bleed readily on contact if you have chronic colitis.

My father gets attacks of acute colitis. What should he do to treat the condition?

He should go to bed, drink plenty of fruit juice, and take kaolin and morphine mixture or codeine to reduce the severity of the diarrhea and pain. If his colitis is the result of an allergic reaction to certain foods, he should try to avoid them.

Colitis is an inflammation of the colon's mucous membrane, and it is unpleasant and debilitating. However, although chronic colitis can become serious, and a long-term problem, acute colitis is usually easy to treat.

The function of the colon is to move solid material from the small intestine to the anus and to absorb salt and water delivered to it from the small intestine. Colitis is an inflammation of the colon's mucous membrane. There are two kinds of colitis. Acute colitis is often a result of an infection or an allergy, and lasts only a short while; chronic, or ulcerative, colitis is much more serious, can have serious complications, and requires prolonged treatment. Chronic colitis is most common in the age group 20 to 40, but can occur at any age. Acute colitis is caused by infections such as amebic and bacillary dysentery; typhoid; enteroviruses; and, most commonly, allergies to certain foods. The cause of chronic colitis is unknown, but there are a few theories. Bacterial infection and allergies to milk and milk products have been cited (see Bacteria). It may also be a result of emotional stress.

In both acute and chronic colitis, the symptoms are abdominal pain, followed by an explosion of watery diarrhea. In chronic colitis, there may be as many as 15 to 20 bowel movements each day. Large quantities of mucus, pus, and sometimes blood are passed with the movements. On occasion there is rectal tenesmus (an ineffectual urge to defecate). In more severe cases dehydration, anemia, loss of appetite and weight, vomiting, and high fever may be present.

For acute colitis, bed rest is advisable. Doses of a kaolin and morphine mixture stop diarrhea. The mainstay of treatment for chronic colitis is salazopyrin (a combination of antibiotic and aspirinlike drugs), taken three times a day. A liquid preparation of hydrocortisone can be given as a suppository; this has a marked soothing effect. Diet should consist of bland, high-protein food, with only a small amount of fruit and roughage (see Diet). Psychotherapy, when the cause is psychological, may help.

With acute colitis, the outlook is excellent as long as the cause of the illness is removed. Some patients recover after a single attack of chronic colitis, but for a greater proportion it may become a fact of life, though one that can be controlled.

See also: Allergies; Anemia; Anus; Diarrhea; Kaolin; Morphine; Vomiting

HOW COLITIS AFFECTS THE BODY

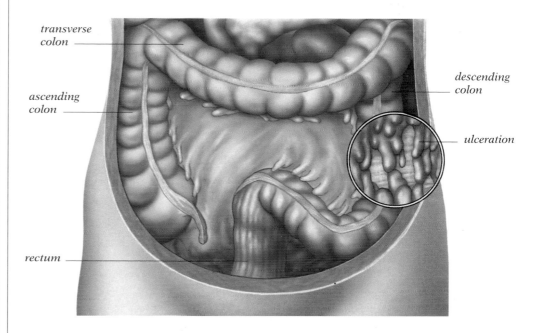

transverse colon

ascending colon

descending colon

ulceration

rectum

▲ *Here, chronic colitis has caused ulcers (inset) in the mucous membrane of the colon.*

Colonic irrigation

This controversial treatment is used by some holistic practitioners for a variety of bowel and other problems. Although the treatment dates from as early as 1500 B.C.E. in Egypt, it has recently gained in popularity once again.

Questions and Answers

What is the difference between colonic irrigation and an enema?

Colonic irrigation is more thorough than an enema, penetrating farther into the bowels and lasting longer. In an enema the water is left in the intestine, but in colonic irrigation there is a constant flow in and out. Enemas tend to be performed by doctors or nurses, whereas colonic irrigation is more likely to be part of holistic medical treatment.

Is the treatment very embarrassing or painful?

The patient wears a special gown designed to preserve as much modesty as possible. There may be slight discomfort when the speculum is inserted, but that is all. Your colon will start to feel full before the water flowing into it is released; this is an unfamiliar, but not unpleasant, sensation. The therapist adjusts the water temperature to a comfortable level.

Is the treatment hygienic?

Yes, if it is properly performed. Equipment is either disposable or disinfected using hospital-approved techniques. The piping system is completely closed so that there is no smell or external contact with the water. The water used is purified or filtered.

Do I need to prepare for the treatment in any way?

Not really. The more relaxed you are, the better it works. You can eat beforehand, but not a large meal. There is no need to rest after the treatment—practitioners say that many people feel instant benefits in terms of more energy and a greater sense of well-being —but you are likely to need to visit the bathroom as soon as the treatment is finished, and you will feel very empty afterward.

The colon is the major part of the large intestine (see Colon and Colitis); it is the last part of the digestive tract, in which the final processes of the digestive system take place (see Digestive System).

In the colon, water and water-soluble nutrients are absorbed, and some vitamins are synthesized. The remaining matter, which consists of toxins, mucus, dead cells from the rest of the digestive system, and indigestible food (roughage), is moved along the colon by the expanding and contracting of its walls (an action called peristalsis) and is gradually dehydrated until it forms a fecal mass. This waste material is then stored in the rectum before being eliminated through the anus as feces (see Anus).

Inner wall

The colon has an inner wall that consists of a mucous membrane designed to absorb liquids. It also produces mucus that lubricates the waste matter and makes it easier for this matter to pass along the colon (see Mucus). If waste matter accumulates on the walls of the colon, the system stops functioning properly. The waste matter builds up in the colon and causes a variety of problems throughout the body.

Colonic irrigation, also known as colonic hydrotherapy or colonic lavage, is a method of cleaning out this accumulated waste matter and helping the colon return to full working order.

Historical techniques

Colonic irrigation is not new. Similar practices were mentioned in 1500 B.C.E. in the ancient Egyptian document Ebers Papyrus, and again by the 16th-century French surgeon Ambroise Paré. Today, with bowel disorders said to affect one in three people in the West and cancer of the colon second only to heart disease as a cause of death, colonic irrigation has become popular once again (see Cancer).

Colonic health

Much of the work done in the colon is carried out with the help of billions of microbes—bacteria, viruses, and fungi. These produce vitamins, break down toxins, and protect us from infection. However, the delicate balance of this internal ecosystem can easily be disturbed by a number of factors, including stress, pollution, drugs, lack of exercise, and the wrong diet.

When this happens, waste matter builds up, restricting the normal activity of the colon, and the problem may get worse over the years. Not only can this cause minor health problems, such as intestinal discomfort, gas, and constipation, but it can also cause more serious ones, such as colitis (chronic inflammation of the bowel), diverticulitis (in which infected sacs appear in the colon), and even cancer.

Toxins

According to holistic therapists, if toxins are not properly broken down and eliminated, they can be reabsorbed by the body (see Holistic Medicine). They can then cause all sorts of problems ranging from headaches and fatigue to frequent bouts of infection, candida, and acne (see Acne

Problems for which colonic irrigation may be prescribed

acne
allergies
arthritis
bloating
candida (thrush)
chronic fatigue
colitis (colonitis)
constipation
Crohn's disease
diarrhea
diverticulitis (diverticulosis)
flatulence (gas)
frequent infection
headaches
hemorrhoids
irritable bowel syndrome (IBS)
itching anus
migraine
stomach pains

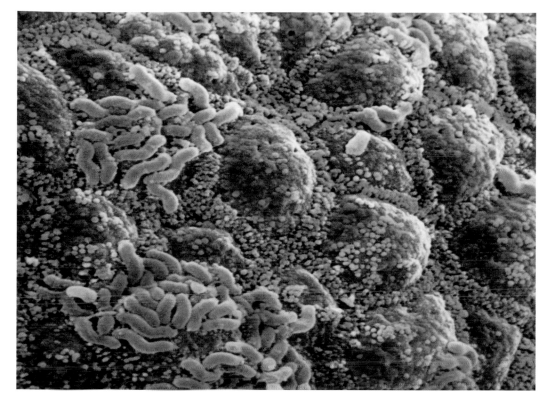

◄ In a healthy colon feces are produced as water, and nutrients are absorbed through the walls of the colon from the digested food passing through it. Problems can arise when an accumulation of waste matter builds up on the walls of the colon, interfering with the absorption process.

A sterile speculum (a kind of surgical instrument that is used for holding open a cavity in the body) is inserted into the rectum, and then water at low pressure is introduced through an inlet tube and fed progressively in waves into the colon while the water, waste, and gas are piped away through another tube—the evacuation tube While this is going on, the therapist will be gently massaging the abdomen to stimulate peristalsis and to promote the evacuation of waste. Afterward

and Pimples). In addition, a buildup of toxins in the body can lead to less specific problems such as lack of sex drive (see Libido) and premature aging.

The unhealthy gut

Colonic irrigation practitioners believe that few people with a modern Western lifestyle have a really healthy gut. Ideally humans should eliminate the contents of the bowels two to three times a day, but many people do not even manage to do so once each day, and some become badly constipated. Diarrhea is another unpleasant problem, caused when food passes too quickly through the body so that much of it is left in the colon (see Diarrhea). The wrong diet can also cause the body to make too much mucus, which can leave behind a gluelike coating on the bowel wall that may then build up and solidify over the years, causing problems in the gut.

The treatment

Most people are referred to a colonic irrigation practitioner by another holistic therapist, such as a naturopath, a homeopath, or a herbalist, in connection with some specific problem. However, even when a specific problem does not exist, practioners of colonic irrigation suggest that their treatment is also a useful therapeutic measure, which can be undergone at the change of the seasons, for instance, or during a period of prolonged stress, such as after a death in the family or the breakup of a marriage. An important part of the first consultation is advice on the correct diet and lifestyle to complement the treatment.

The procedure

The actual irrigation itself takes from half to three-quarters of an hour. Having changed into a special gown and having had the process explained in detail, the individual will be asked to lie flat on the treatment table and relax.

the patient may be given a suppository-type implant made either of herbs, to help loosen the accumulated waste, or of microbes, to help reestablish the gut's healthy ecosystem (see Suppositories).

Frequency of treatments

The number of treatments a patient will need depends on how long the problem or problems have existed, how severe they are, and how relaxed an individual is during the treatment. The efforts that the patient makes regarding diet and exercise to back up the treatment are also taken into account.

Some people may only need one session, but others may require several, with follow-up sessions at widely spaced intervals over the course of, say, a year. Initially the usual recommended number is four to six, at weekly intervals.

The conventional view

Some doctors believe that colonic irrigation can bring temporary relief for a range of ailments, but that it is not a long-term cure. Others believe that it is simply a useless form of quackery or that prolonged use of colonic irrigation can weaken the body's natural ability to expel feces, and that, at worst, the practice is dangerous.

Certified practitioners

Because colonic irrigation is a fairly controversial treatment, it is important to make sure that the therapist carrying out the treatment is reputable, fully trained, and experienced in a body-based holistic therapy. He or she could even be a relatively conventional practitioner, such as a nurse or doctor. At the very least it is important that the practitioner has a thorough knowledge of anatomy and physiology.

See also: **Bacteria; Constipation; Crohn's disease; Diet; Diverticulitis; Feces; Flatulence; Hemorrhoids; Rectum; Viruses**

Colonoscopy

The ability to directly examine the interior of most of the large intestine provides doctors with a valuable tool for the early detection and diagnosis of a range of important conditions, including cancer.

Questions and Answers

I have to have a colonoscopy. Are there any dangers?

Millions of colonoscopies are done each year, and complications are rare. There is a very small risk of perforation of the wall of the colon. If a tissue sample (biopsy) is taken, there is a possibility that you may see some blood in the next bowel movement. This will do no harm, but if you have any abnormal bleeding tendency you must tell your doctor.

Is it a good idea to have a routine colonoscopy at regular intervals?

Colorectal cancer is so common, and early diagnosis so important, that many doctors believe that everyone around 40 should have a colonoscopy. The problem is really economic. Other screening tests also compete for attention. If you have a history of colonic polyps, you need frequent checks.

Several of my relatives have developed colon cancer. Should I have a colonoscopy?

Yes. There are some familial conditions that make it more likely for colon cancer to develop, and colonoscopy can detect these. You should bear in mind, however, that when any disease is common in a population it is statistically likely to occur frequently in a family, without any genetic basis.

Is colonoscopy more difficult to perform on women than on men?

Difficulty is experienced in about 30 percent of women but only in about 16 percent of men, because women have a longer colon, especially in the transverse part. Diverticulitis produces inflamed pouches protruding from the wall of the colon. This may make colonoscopy difficult in either sex.

Until the development of what are called endoscopic methods, doctors had to diagnose conditions on the basis of the patient's history, the symptoms, and the clinical signs, helped in some cases by X rays and scans (see Diagnostic Imaging). While these are still important parts of the clinical examination, the ability to make direct visual inspection of the actual diseased areas has substantially increased the accuracy and speed of diagnosis. Colonoscopy is the use of endoscopic methods to examine the inside of the large intestine, the colon. It has, to a large extent, replaced the barium enema as a diagnostic procedure (see Barium Liquids).

Colonoscopy is done using a steerable, flexible, fiberoptic colonoscope. This instrument consists of a cable about 39 inches (1 m) long attached to a control head. The cable looks deceptively simple but actually contains several distinct channels, along which pass fiberoptic bundles for internal illumination and viewing, specially designed instruments for taking biopsy samples (see Biopsy), and fluid for washing the area under view. In spite of this complexity, the endoscope cable is flexible and the tip can be turned in any direction so that it can be moved along the interior of the colon to allow direct visual inspection of the entire route. Control knobs in the head of the instrument allow the operator to change the curvature and direction of the tip. The head also includes the eyepiece for the operator and the openings for the various channels. The instrument is usually fitted with a color video camera and viewed on a computer monitor. This allows the convenient taking of color photographs, which are stored on the computer for reference.

COLONOSCOPY

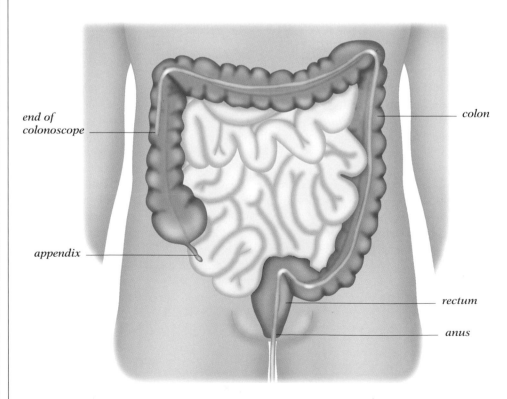

end of colonoscope

colon

appendix

rectum

anus

▲ *During a colonoscopy, a flexible tube is inserted into the anus, through the rectum, and into the colon, which can then be viewed for the presence of polyps or other disorders.*

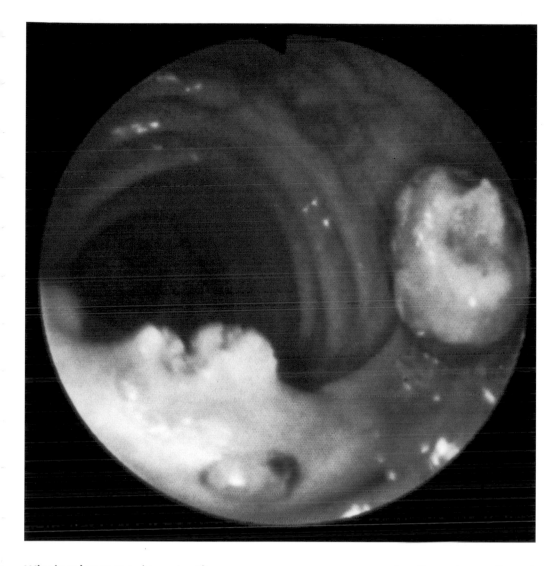

◄ *A colonoscopy shows up two white polyps, which can usually be removed using a diathermic snare during the procedure.*

principal importance and advantage of colonoscopy, however, is early diagnosis of colon cancer. If it is identified at an early stage and treated, the outlook is excellent. For this reason, whenever a person notices rectal bleeding that is not due to a minor condition such as piles, colonoscopy is essential. After direct visual examination, the second great advantage of colonoscopy is the ability to take a biopsy. A range of biopsy tools is available, including cup-shaped biopsy forceps, mouse-tooth forceps, alligator forceps, and wire loop snare. All these can be controlled and used under direct vision through the endoscope.

How is colonoscopy done?

Different doctors may have different routines for colonoscopy, but the following procedure is typical. Two days before the procedure the patient is started on a low-residue diet. This is a diet that is almost wholly absorbed so as to reduce the amount of stools. The day before, morning and evening doses of a laxative such as sodium picosulfate are given, and on that day only a light lunch followed by clear fluids is allowed. On the day of the examination the patient is allowed clear fluids only.

Why is colonoscopy important?

Colonoscopy can provide direct and clear indication of the causes of unexplained bleeding from the bowel, unexplained pain in the lower abdomen, or long-term and persistent diarrhea. It is an excellent way of detecting inflammation of the bowel wall and of determining the cause of the inflammation. Colon-wall ulceration is also a sign of certain diseases, and colonoscopy can detect the ulcers and possibly establish the full diagnosis. Colonic polyps are immediately obvious and can be removed (see Polyps). The

Colonoscopy does not require a general anesthetic but is nearly always done under sedation. A sedative such as a benzodiazepine with a painkiller such as demerol (meperidine) is given by intravenous injection shortly before the examination starts (see Sedatives). This produces calm relaxation and an almost complete absence of pain. The oxygen levels of the blood are monitored during the examination. The tip of the cable of the instrument is passed in through the lubricated anus, producing no more sensation than a normal bowel movement. It is then passed up through the rectum and descending colon, turned across the transverse colon, and down the ascending colon as far as the point at which the small intestine ends. During this passage, the whole of the wall of the colon is inspected all around. Particular attention is paid to the angles (flexures) at which the bowel bends sharply, since the tip tends to pass more quickly at these points. Biopsies are taken of any suspicious areas for pathological examination, and polyps may be snared off and taken for checking.

Conditions for which colonoscopy may be valuable

Amebic dysentery
Cancer of the colon or rectum
Chronic constipation
Crohn's disease
Diverticulitis
Polyposis syndromes
Rectal or colonic polyps
Ulcerative colitis (colonoscopy is avoided in the acute stage)
Unexplained diarrhea
Unexplained rectal bleeding

See also: Cancer; Colon and colitis; Constipation; Crohn's disease; Diarrhea; Endoscopy; Laxatives; Ulcers

Color blindness

Color blindness is a fairly common condition in which those affected have a problem differentiating between certain colors. It occurs more often in men than in women. Color blindness is rarely a serious disadvantage.

Color blindness does not affect the ability to see color, only the ability to distinguish between certain colors. It should not affect your child's learning to read, though in schools where math is taught by using colored bricks, it may cause confusion. If you think your son may be color-blind, take him to an optometrist to have him tested.

If you are male and color blindness runs in your family, then you might be. Perhaps some of the colors on paint charts all look the same to you, or a chance remark from someone has implied that he or she can distinguish between shades that you can't. A test by a set of Ishihara cards, the most common color-blindness test, will indicate if you are color-blind. The cards have bold numerals printed on them in dots of various tints, set against a background of dots of a different hue. If you can't read the numerals, you may be color-blind. These tests are not infallible, however, as some color-blind people can differentiate between the different colored surfaces.

Tobacco and alcohol do not cause color blindness alone but can lead to a gradual deterioration in all aspects of vision. Alcoholism can cause blindness in severe cases. Methyl alcohol, found in methylated spirits, can lead to rapid, permanent blindness. Smokers of very strong tobacco mixtures may have foggy vision, especially if they also drink heavily, but today's more refined tobacco makes this effect a rarity.

Color blindness is the inability to distinguish between different colors. The most common form involves the confusion of red and green. Occasionally , blue and yellow shades are also confused, but this form of color blindness is more difficult to discern, since there are no commonly available tests for it. In rarer forms, all colors are seen as black and white.

Color blindness is very common: about 1 in 20 men and 1 in 200 women are affected. Many people are unaware that they are color-blind until they have their eyes tested by an optometrist.

Most cases of color blindness are hereditary. Women can transmit red-green color blindness as carriers of the gene, without themselves being affected. They can have red-green color blindness only if their father had it and their mother was a carrier. The rare forms affect both sexes equally. Color blindness can also skip a generation and show up in grandchildren.

Causes

The causes of color blindness are unknown. Color is perceived by certain cells, called cones, in the retina of the eye. These contain pigments (coloring matter), which determine the color certain cones will respond to. In the inherited form, color blindness may be due to a lack of one of these pigments.

Sometimes color blindness can occur because of a disease of the retina or optic nerve (the nerve connecting the retina to the brain; see Optic Nerve). This rarer form of color blindness is progressive and associated with a general deterioration of vision. By contrast, in the inherited form the ability to see detail is unaffected and the condition never worsens.

Symptoms

In the common, inherited form, the red-green color-blind person sees the colors red and green as the same hue, the two colors being distinguished only by their intensity. Because the condition is present from birth, people suffering from this form of color blindness have to learn gradually to associate certain tones, textures, and intensities with what people of normal vision see as red and green. In the extremely rare form of total color blindness, perception is monochrome with white shading through various grays, to black, as in early black-and-white television.

Employment problems

Color blindness is not a handicap to everyday life, but when someone's job depends on information conveyed by color, it could become a barrier to employment. Careers in areas such as graphic design and color photography would obviously be unsuitable. Any job that involves reading color-coded maps might also cause problems for a color-blind person.

Red and green are the universal colors for stop and go, and port and starboard, so engine drivers and sailors should not be color-blind. But traffic lights can be distinguished by the position of the lights, so color blindness is not a bar to driving.

Diagnosis

Many people who are color-blind are unaware that they have the condition, particularly if they work in an occupation or live in an environment in which color is not a vital issue. However, the condition may gradually be revealed as the color-blind person discusses the nature of colors with other people and begins to realize that his or her recognition or identification of colors is somewhat different from that of other people.

Any person who suspects that he or she may be color-blind should see a optometrist, who will carry out some form of diagnostic test for color blindness (see Optometrist). The tests usually consist of simple patterns or plates in which numerals can be detected from a group of dots. Most people who are color-blind will be unable to see, or decipher, the correct number and will tend to interpret the color of the numeral and the background dots as the same.

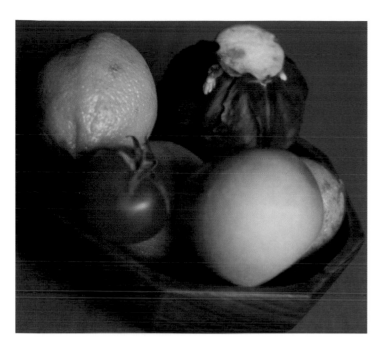 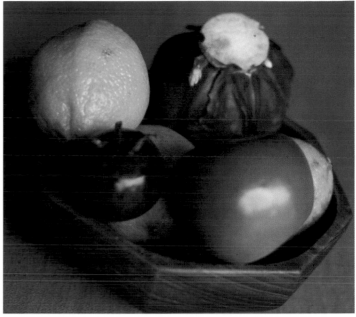

▲ *A person with normal color vision would see the fruits and vegetables pictured above as they appear on the left. A person with red-green color blindness, however, would perceive them as they appear on the right.*

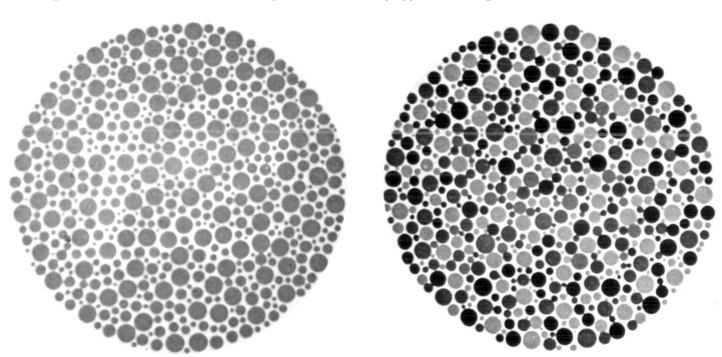

▲ *Almost everyone can distinguish the number 12 against the background in the figure on the left—the first of a series of cards used to test for color blindness. When looking at the figure on the right, however, if someone cannot see the dark red 9 he or she is green-blind, and if someone cannot see the lighter red 6, he or she is red-blind.*

Treatment and outlook

There is no cure for inherited color blindness. However, the weakening of vision associated with a diseased retina or optic nerve may be improved or arrested, so a person who notices that his or her ability to discriminate between colors is worsening should see a doctor.

Inherited color blindness is a harmless condition of which many people are unaware, although it may prohibit a person from entering certain occupations. However, most color-blind people will learn to compensate for the condition and may even find that they are able to discern details and images that normally sighted people cannot. For example, the U.S. Army has found that color-blind people can easily spot camouflage colors, which escape the detection of normally sighted people.

See also: **Eyes and eyesight; Genetic diseases and disorders; Retina and retinal disorders**

Color therapy

Is color therapy a belief system, and can it work even if you do not believe in the presence of the aura?

Exposure to different colors causes very subtle molecular changes to the cells, so it is not necessary to believe in the aura to reap the benefits. However, having an open mind helps, as color therapy works gradually. You may be instructed to do certain things, such as visualize a color, wear or surround yourself with particular colors, or make your own solarized water.

Is color therapy the same thing as art therapy?

There are a number of similarities. Meditation and contemplation of a work of art are used in color therapy, but the body and mind are treated through the aura, whereas art therapy focuses on the painting or sculpture that the client creates and on the relationship between client and therapist. Color therapy is used to heal physical illness, whereas art therapy treats only the unconscious aspects of illness. Both therapies, however, aim to bring unconscious feelings to a conscious level, where they can be explored with the therapist. In art therapy the technical ability to draw is of much less importance than the expression and exploration of unconscious feelings.

Can I use color therapy techniques on myself?

Yes, much can be gained from self-therapy if you have an adequate understanding of the powers of color. At first, however, it is better to learn from a qualified therapist. The aura is delicate and complex, so it can be adversely affected by over- or understimulation with color. A color therapist may also suggest beneficial color choices for clothes and the colors used for paint and fabrics in rooms in which you live and work.

Color therapy is an ancient healing technique that is still important today in Ayurvedic medicine in India. Practitioners use color therapy to balance a person's energy, wherever it is lacking.

Color therapy encompasses many different practices. Stained glass, solarized water, oils enriched with color, gemstones, and crystals are all used to harness the subtle energies and vibrations of light and color. Color therapy may alleviate many health problems and harmonize people's natural rhythms and energies.

Electromagnetic spectrum

Visible color is only a part of the electromagnetic spectrum. From one end of the spectrum to the other, through radio waves (which cannot be seen), infrared rays, visible rays, ultraviolet light, X rays, gamma rays, and cosmic rays, the frequencies become higher and the waves shorter. Most rays are invisible to the human eye but are used in scientific and medical applications.

Visible light, which is made up of eight colors, is in the middle of the spectrum. Each color is a form of radiation with its own vibrational frequency. Color therapy uses all the colors of this spectrum, their vibrational forces being manipulated to cause molecular changes at a cellular level. Each cell in the body can be affected by color, so that even blind people may benefit from this type of therapy.

▲ *Complementary colors: those opposite each other are used together.*

The whole person

A person is said to be made up of body, mind, and spirit, which must work together in harmony for his or her well-being. The body's cells and organs are in continual movement, causing vibrational frequencies akin to those of color and sound. Color therapists believe they can see colors in the aura. If colors become fuzzy and unclear, there may be a problem in mind, body, or spirit, or all three.

The aura

The aura is an invisible cloak around the body, consisting of multicolored electromagnetic light energy with several layers, each radiating its own color. The aura absorbs white light and then directs its different vitalizing rays around the body. Color therapy identifies areas of disharmony,

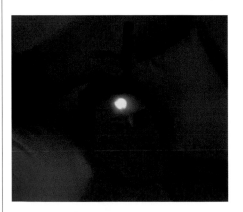

▲ *A therapist projects a light onto the patient's frontal chakra in a room lit with a complementary color.*

Reflexology, followed by applications of color to problem sites, can be a very powerful and therapeutic technique.

Yoga, used with a good knowledge of color, is effective for harmonizing the physical body. Techniques in use include color breathing, visualization, and meditation.

Gemstones resonate sounds and colors and their healing properties can be harnessed by placing the stones in patterns on the body.

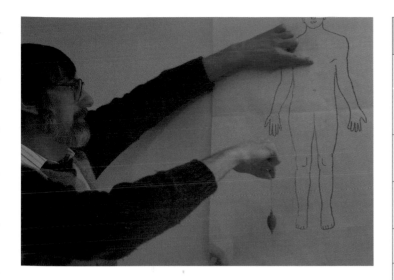

▲ *In this method of color therapy a chart of the human body is bathed in a color complementary to the healing color before the patient is exposed to therapeutic colors in a treatment room.*

and finds the colors that are needed to retune a person's aura. The aura has seven energy centers called chakras, each with its own color and linked to a gland in the endocrine system and certain physical organs.

Types of color therapy
Aura-soma color therapy draws on aspects of aromatherapy, herbal medicine, and mineral supplementation. The patient is asked to select four bottles of dual-colored healing oils from a range of 95 different color combinations, such as gold over yellow or blue over green, which together make up a glimmering rainbow of color. The system hinges on the belief that a person is naturally drawn to the colors that reflect his or her own individual needs for healing .

The therapist interprets the patient's color selection, identifying the characteristics of the soul and spirit in the first bottle; childhood and the recent past in the second; the patient's current state in the third; and the energies that are drawing toward the person in the fourth. The colors missing from the selection also have significance. The therapist may recommend a special preparation, such as a color-enriched healing oil, for application to the body and relevant chakra area.

Hygeia color therapy uses colored (qualified) light sent through stained glass. It starts with a counseling session before the patient is asked to sign along the back of a chart representing the human spine—the central column of energy linking the brain to the body's organs. Using the energies conveyed through the signature, the therapist dowses each vertebra with a pendulum to find hidden problems.

After the therapist decides which colors are needed, the patient may be treated in various ways. The patient may be asked to put on a white gown and enter a treatment room, where he or she will be subjected to a sequence of carefully timed exposures to colored lights. Sometimes small stained-glass filters are used to concentrate color on a particular area of the body. For example, a turquoise filter may be used to treat an infected finger, and a green filter to treat a cyst.

The patient may also be given solarized water—simple spring water that has been encased in a filter of colored glass and exposed to sunlight in order to change its chemical makeup. Red glass will make the water taste sour and is used to provide energy; under blue glass, water will taste sweet and promote relaxation. Water solarized

Colors, their meaning, and their uses

NINE MAJOR COLORS OF VISIBLE LIGHT

Red: strength, energy, sexuality, power, alertness; for low blood pressure, lethargy, impotence

Orange: joy, independence; for depression, muscle cramps, and spasms, and to lower blood pressure

Yellow: intellect, objectivity, critical thinking, reason; for rheumatism and arthritis, and to aid digestion

Green: harmony, balance; for cleansing purposes, cancer

Turquoise: purity, calmness; for inflammation, AIDS/HIV, tension

Blue: relaxation, peace, expansion, growth; for high blood pressure, stress, asthma, migraine, burns

Violet: dignity, honor, hope; for lack of self-esteem, infection

Magenta: release, meditation; for change, freedom

White light (all of the above): innocence, isolation, wisdom; for clarity, neutrality, as a diuretic, and as an emotional stabilizer

PIGMENT COLORS

Black: depth; for attracting humility

Gray: dedication; for pride (rarely used)

Brown: dedication, commitment; for selfishness (rarely used)

with yellow is used for arthritic conditions, green for cleansing, and turquoise for strengthening the immune system. The healing power of these waters is very gentle, and the results will thus not be felt immediately. Solarized creams can be used in a similar way.

Color in clothing and the home
Color therapists believe that using colors in clothing and the home can enhance a person's comfort and well-being. For example, people sensitive to the cold should wear red, particularly on the hands and feet, as even looking at that color can make people feel warmer. Yet a color is best balanced with its complementary color for the most benefit. Before choosing colors in the home, a room's function and size should be considered. A room will seem smaller if it has a lot of red, orange, or yellow, and larger with blue, white, or indigo. Green maintains proportions and is considered good for cardiac circulation, but too much is tiring. Red is powerful and may overstimulate the nerves and ego. Blue is calming and helps expand the mind.

See also: **Alternative medicine**

Colostomy

A colostomy is performed when there is an obstruction in the colon, or following surgical treatment for cancer. Despite having to wear a colostomy bag, an individual can live a full life.

A colostomy is a surgical opening made in the front of the abdominal wall. Feces (waste material from the colon, which is the major part of the large intestine) can be passed out from this opening instead of taking the usual route via the rectum. The operation is performed when, after surgery on the colon, it has been found impossible or impracticable to restore the normal internal continuity of the bowel (see Colon and Colitis). Colostomy may be necessary to relieve colonic obstruction, but it is most commonly a sequel to removal of a cancerous segment of the bowel.

Site of colostomy

The location of the problem in the colon determines the type of surgical procedure that is performed and the position of the colostomy. Colostomies performed on the right side of the colon open on the right side of the abdomen and discharge liquid feces. Those performed on the left side open on the left side of the pelvis, and they pass much more solid material; this is because more liquid has been absorbed from the food during digestion by the time it has reached this part of the colon.

LEFT-SIDE COLOSTOMY

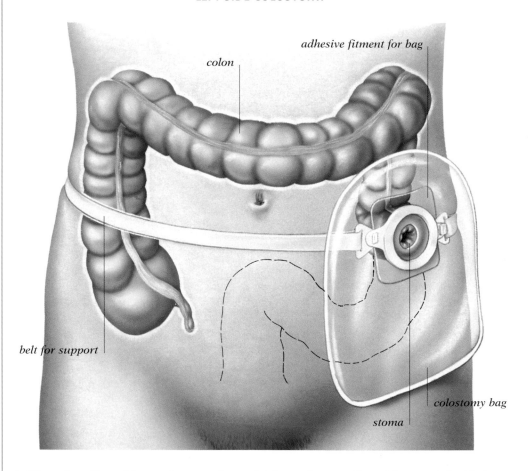

colon

adhesive fitment for bag

belt for support

colostomy bag

stoma

▲ *Waste is collected in a colostomy bag, which can be on either side. In a left-sided colostomy, feces are solid and the bag does not have to be worn constantly. The belt provides extra security at night.*

▶ *A travel kit for care of the stoma (opening) contains all that is needed for changing a colostomy bag discreetly when a person is away from home.*

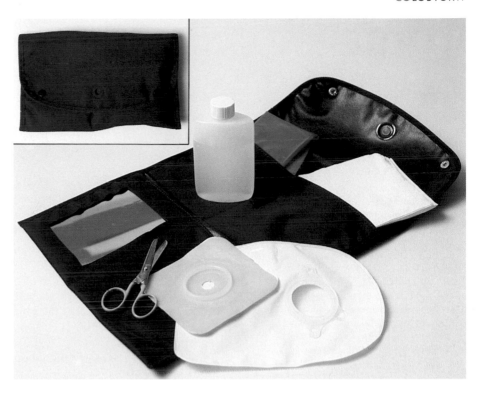

Why is it done?

A colostomy is undertaken only when there is no other method of allowing the colonic contents to be expelled. Most often the operation is necessary following cancer surgery, but it is also performed to treat other bowel diseases, such as ulcerative colitis. Tumors that develop high up in the colon may be dealt with simply by removing the affected part of the colon and joining the two ends together. When the tumor grows close to the rectum, this cannot be done, and a colostomy is performed in the left side of the abdomen. When the whole length of the colon is diseased, an opening is made on the right side.

Coping with a colostomy

The method of dealing with a colostomy depends on the site where the opening was made. Right-sided colostomies discharge liquid matter continually. A drainage bag must be worn at all times, and there is no control over when the opening will discharge.

Left-sided colostomies, on the other hand, produce solid material, because there is more colon available to absorb water from the feces. After things have settled down following surgery, most people discharge their feces once or twice every 24 hours, often just before or after breakfast. Others have their major movement after the evening meal, but in any one individual the colostomy functions at around the same time each day. Most physicians and surgeons suggest using a colostomy bag for solid material; with practice, this bag can be worn just in the morning or evening. The colostomy wound tends to close up, and people are taught to prevent this by gently inserting a clean finger into the opening once a week.

The importance of diet

The greatest enemy of someone with a colostomy is diarrhea. Loose stools cause the colostomy to function irregularly, and this can be embarrassing. Certain foods are known to cause this sort of trouble, particularly uncooked vegetables, fruit, whole wheat bread, cereal, beer, and certain types of wine. Most people are able to identify the particular type of food that causes them trouble and can avoid it.

Medication may be given to slow down the action of the colon, thus allowing more water to be absorbed. Commonly used products that increase the bulk of the feces are methylcellulose or kaolin (see Kaolin). Drugs derived from opium, such as codeine, are efficient at slowing down the action of the colon.

Offensive-smelling gas can sometimes be a problem, but this can also be avoided by not eating certain foods—and most people know the things that disagree with them—or by taking a supplement that sweetens the odor (see Flatulence).

Outlook

A colostomy operation does not shorten a person's life, and an opening in the abdominal wall does not make him or her more prone to infection. The greatest difficulty is in coming to terms with the disability. It is not unusual for a period of depression to follow surgery of this type and the patient may find it helpful to talk to someone who has had a colostomy for some time.

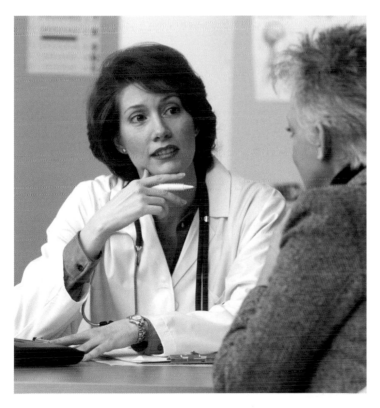

▲ *The most important thing after having a colostomy is to come to terms with it and to continue living as before.*

See also: **Cancer; Feces; Surgery**

Coma

Questions and Answers

In medical shows on television, unconscious patients are often sent for a CT scan. What is this for?

Computerized tomographic scanning, also called computerized axial tomography (CT or CAT) scanning, is a technique used to produce two-dimensional images of the brain (or other parts of the body). For a CT scan of the brain, the patient lies on a table with his or her head inside the scanner. The scanner rotates around the head, taking X rays from many angles. A computer reconstructs the images as slices through the brain. The slices show internal structures more clearly than a normal X ray and can be used to tell if there is brain damage or a tumor.

Is persistent vegetative state the same as a coma?

Patients with severe brain damage often make a slow but steady recovery. In some cases, however, this stops after some initial improvement. If the patient remains unconscious without further improvement but is able to breathe without a mechanical ventilator, the condition is known as a persistent vegetative state. The patient will be fed, usually by a stomach tube, and given treatment to prevent the formation of pressure sores. Patients may stay alive in this state for years.

Why do some patients have their life support machines turned off?

If permanent damage has occurred to the centers in the brain stem that control breathing, heart rate, and temperature, the patient is said to be brain-dead. Once a patient is certified as brain-dead, life support is often withdrawn, as there is no chance of recovery—even if treatment were continued, the heart would stop within a few days. The equipment may then be used to save another patient's life.

The deep, sleeplike state of unconsciousness is the result of certain changes that have occurred in the brain. The causes and severity vary, but in its most extreme form—the coma—it may be very long-lasting.

The brain is far more complex than even the most advanced computer. Linked with the peripheral nervous system, it controls all of a person's movements and bodily processes, such as breathing, heartbeat, and digestion, as well as the senses and functions like speech, memory, and intelligence.

Different areas of the brain control different functions, and there are a number of critical areas, including the cerebral cortex, the thalamus, the brain stem, and a group of cells within the brain stem called the reticular formation, that play an important part in maintaining consciousness itself. If anything causes changes in these key areas—for example, if a person receives a severe blow to the head that results in bleeding in the brain, or if there is an illness or some form of poisoning that alters the chemical balance of the brain—then the individual may become unconscious.

Losing consciousness

If a person becomes unconscious, the electrical activity of his or her brain changes. This activity can be measured using a machine called an electroencephalograph, or EEG (see Electroencephalogram). Special electrodes are attached to the skin on the scalp and connected by wires to the machine. The brain's electrical impulses are shown as a pattern of waves, which varies according to the degree

▼ *This coma patient is able to breath by himself, and his eyes are partially open.*

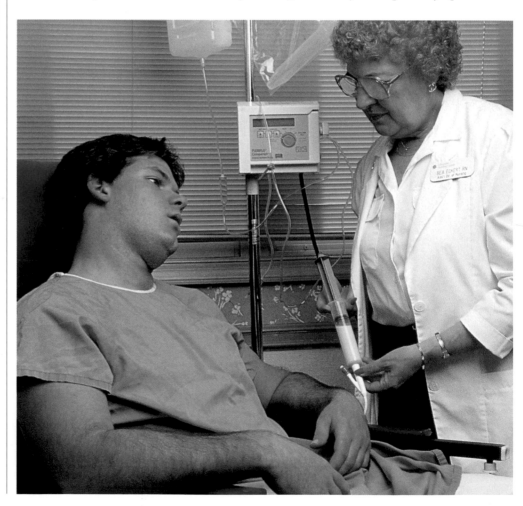

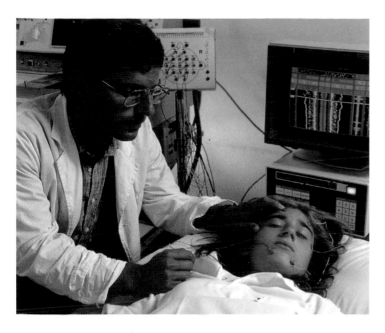

▲ *The electroencephalogram (EEG) records the electrical activity of the brain of coma patients through differences in readings from electrodes attached to the scalp.*

of alertness or unconsciousness. During unconsciousness the pattern is very slow, with about three waves per second. When someone is coming around from unconsciousness—or awakening from sleep—the waves start to increase in frequency until the pattern is rapid and jagged at full consciousness (see Sleep and Sleep Problems).

Unconsciousness is a sleeplike state, but it is much deeper than sleep. An unconscious person will be completely unaware of his or her surroundings and will not respond to external stimuli, such as noise. In some cases (for example, a concussion following a blow to the head), unconsciousness lasts for just a few seconds, but in its most extreme form it may last for many weeks, and the sufferer is said to be in a coma.

A coma is a very serious condition. It affects the activity of the whole brain; and even reflex actions, such as coughing and tendon reflexes (the type of reflex experienced when a physician hits the knee with a tendon hammer), are absent. A person in the very deepest coma may not respond even to the most painful stimuli.

Major causes of coma

The most common causes of coma are a period of loss of blood to the brain; poisoning, bleeding (hemorrhage) in the brain, a brain tumor, shock, and bacterial blood poisoning.

A severe blow to the head may rupture one or more blood vessels, causing a hemorrhage. Another common cause of hemorrhage is stroke. Most people who suffer strokes are over 65, but strokes can happen at any age, especially in people with high blood pressure (see Stroke). Whatever the cause, a brain hemorrhage can rapidly lead to unconsciousness and, if the bleeding is severe, to coma.

Brain tumors, both benign and malignant, can eventually lead to a state of coma (see Tumors). Because the bones of the skull make it impossible for any type of tumor to expand outward, the soft brain tissue is dangerously compressed as the tumor gets bigger. Unless it is treated, there will be permanent brain damage, and if the affected area is one of those that control consciousness, the sufferer will go into a coma and then die.

In the condition known as shock, the circulatory system collapses; once this happens the blood supply to all the vital organs, including the brain, is reduced. When the brain is no longer receiving enough blood, the collection of symptoms called shock syndrome will become apparent. These include sweating, blurred vision, rapid breathing, and faintness that can lead to unconsciousness and coma. This type of shock can be brought on by massive internal or external bleeding, heart attacks, and loss of body fluid caused by various illnesses, such as cholera (see Shock).

Someone who has been poisoned by fumes, chemicals, or drugs may become comatose. Some drugs, such as barbiturates, depress the activity of the brain stem, one of the parts of the brain controlling consciousness. An overdose of this type of drug will therefore cause unconsciousness and, unless it is quickly treated, a coma.

Carbon monoxide poisoning (which can be caused by inhaling an excessive amount of fumes from an automobile or another vehicle) can result in a coma because it reduces the amount of oxygen in the blood, leading to an oxygen deficiency in the tissues of the brain.

Other causes

Two other causes of comas are untreated diabetes (a disease caused by a deficiency in insulin produced in the pancreas) and hypothyroidism (a disease caused by underactivity of the thyroid gland, which causes all chemical processes in the body to slow down).

A diabetic coma results when the body uses fat instead of glucose to provide energy, and poisonous acids called ketones form as a by-product (see Diabetes). This can happen to a person before his or her diabetes has been diagnosed or treated, or if treatment is neglected. An overdose of insulin, leading to very low blood sugar, can also cause a coma (see Insulin). This is called hypoglycemic coma, and it calls for urgent administration of sugar, or an injection of glucagon, to save life. People who suffer from hypothyroidism may go into a coma brought on by cold weather or certain drugs, especially some types of sedative.

Some infections can also cause a coma. Most of these are viral (see Viruses). The virus can spread to the nervous system and brain from an infection such as mumps, measles, glandular fever, herpes simplex, or HIV, causing inflammation of the brain cells, or encephalitis. In most cases the infection causes only encephalitis and not subsequent coma.

Treatment

The treatment of a coma depends on the initial cause. If it has been caused by bleeding, surgery may be needed to release trapped blood or clots, relieve the pressure on the brain, and repair the damaged blood vessels. It may also be possible to remove part or all of a brain tumor with surgery, and this may be followed by radiotherapy to kill remaining tumor cells (see Radiotherapy).

Until recently, if a coma lasted for more than 24 hours, it usually resulted in some form of permanent brain damage (see Brain Damage and Disease). Nowadays a life-support system can take over vital brain functions such as maintaining blood pressure and breathing, allowing time for treatment to succeed and natural healing to occur. The longer a coma lasts, however, the less chance there is of a complete recovery.

See also: **Blood poisoning; Brain; Brain death; Cholera; Hemorrhage; Memory; Nervous system; Poisoning; Thyroid; Unconsciousness**

Common cold

The common cold affects millions of people every year, particularly in the winter months. Although research continues, so far no cure for the common cold has ever been found.

Questions and Answers

I've often been tempted to try cold cures that I see in advertisements. Do these work?

There is no cure for a cold. Some commercial products contain antihistamines, which can reduce secretions and help you sleep. But a cold will always run its course.

My father always seems to have more colds in the summer than in the winter. Why is this?

He may have hay fever, which has symptoms similar to those of the cold virus. Such allergic reactions are usually seasonal, except when someone becomes allergic to material that is present in the air all year long, such as house dust. In such cases it can be difficult, without tests, to distinguish between an allergy and a cold.

Are there any special foods I can eat to protect myself from colds?

Some people feel that taking large amounts of vitamin C, contained in citrus fruits or ascorbic acid preparations, provides some protection—thus the old belief in honey-and-lemon mixture. However, experiments have not yet proved that this helps.

I've heard that you can get a cold by standing in a draft. Is this true?

No. But exposure to wet and miserable weather may lower your resistance, making it easier for the cold virus to gain entry.

What is the difference between a cold and the flu?

Flu involves a specific virus, whereas a cold involves many different viruses. Flu and colds both have upper respiratory symptoms, but flu symptoms are more severe.

The common cold is not one disease, but many. They all have similar symptoms, all of which are caused by viruses that are transmitted to other people by hand contact, coughing, or sneezing.

Causes

There are at least 150 types of viruses that are known to produce the common cold. Antibiotics are of no use in treatment, nor are there yet any effective antiviral drugs.

Not only is the body faced with a bewildering variety of viruses, but these viruses are always likely to undergo DNA mutations, and no practical solution has yet been found to this very complex problem (see Genetics).

People at risk

The sick, the elderly, and the undernourished are not as good as healthy people at fighting infection, and so they are more susceptible to the ravages of the common cold. Young children, whose immune system has not come into contact with so many viruses (see Immune System), can suffer 20 or more such infections each year—as often happens when children start school.

Symptoms and dangers

The symptoms of the common cold are well known. The first sign is a feeling of being under the weather, which lasts a few hours. This is usually characterized by aching joints and a cold, shivery feeling (see Shivering). The body temperature is commonly subnormal at this stage; within the next few days—and sometimes hours—the body temperature goes up. A person may have a sore throat and generally feel miserable. As the throat begins to clear, the eyes and nose begin to stream, and there are bouts of repeated sneezing. For most people the common cold is a relatively trivial illness, lasting only a few days. However, it can be a serious matter for a person who suffers from bronchitis, especially if he or she is also a smoker (see Bronchitis).

Treatment

Unless complications like bronchitis develop, there is no need to call a doctor. The best plan is to make the patient as comfortable as possible. Acetaminophen or aspirin can help reduce a fever. Aspirin should not be given to children with viral infections—acetaminophen is safer.

▼▲ *Colds are caused by many viruses, including the coronavirus (below), and the symptoms of a cold are very unpleasant (above).*

See also: **Aspirin and analgesics; Coughing; Fevers; Infection and infectious diseases; Joints; Nose; Sneezing; Sore throat; Temperature; Viruses**

Complexes and compulsions

Is avoiding the cracks in the sidewalk always an example of compulsive behavior?

In children it's more of a game, but if the child believes too strongly that something terrible will happen if he or she steps on the cracks, the resulting anxiety may cause the game to become a compulsion. In adults it is a fairly harmless compulsion.

Do short men always have an inferiority complex?

By no means. But they may tend more than tall men to have this complex because they get pushed around more, especially when they are young. It would also be true to say that small men with a natural tendency toward anxiety are more likely to have an inferiority complex than others who are both taller and more relaxed in disposition. But a tall man can also have an inferiority complex.

Are children of one-parent families likely to have a complex?

Not particularly. Of course, since one-parent families are often under greater stress than two-parent families, the children can be more susceptible to complexes. Such families, however have more practice at coping successfully with stress, and children will be better at growing out of complexes.

How can I stop overeating? Is overeating compulsive behavior?

Overeating may be due not to a compulsion but to an upset metabolism. If this is not so, your behavior may be a compulsion, or it may be a displacement activity in which you compensate for feeling insecure, unloved, or neglected. A doctor, and perhaps a specialist, will help determine the best treatment.

What exactly is a complex or a compulsion? And what should a person do if he or she suffers from one? Because complexes and compulsions are generally caused by anxiety, the solution is to relieve the cause of the worry.

In psychology, a complex is a set of memories and emotions that are strongly linked together (see Psychology). They are often frightening, and they have their origin in childhood, when the world seemed fearsome. If they last into adulthood, they may produce compulsive behavior. This is an attempt to relieve the buildup of anxiety that is the result of the complex; thus the words "complex" and "compulsion" are often linked (see Anxiety). Excessive hand washing is a common example of compulsive behavior, which can become a problem in its own right. The psychiatrist Carl Jung called his psychoanalytical approach the "psychology of complexes." He regarded a complex as a set of ideas containing strong and perhaps frightening emotions that may be repressed and thus barely remembered. A mother complex, for example, is one in which a boy becomes overwhelmed by the fear of a dominating mother and cannot form relationships in adulthood with women he sees as overbearing. However, the misery produced by these problems can be lessened. Compulsions can be removed, and complexes can be treated by psychotherapy. Psychiatry has given names to a large number of these bundles of associated memories, beliefs, attitudes, and acts, many of which have passed into everyday use (see Psychiatry).

Oedipus complex

Almost everyone, for example, has heard of the Oedipus complex, regarded by Sigmund Freud and his followers as a young boy's wish for some form of sexual relationship with his mother and the consequent wish to kill his father out of jealousy. Freud was of the opinion that every male child has this complex for some period during infancy and that it needed to be resolved (grown out of) before further adult emotional development could take place. The castration complex, according to Freud, follows the Oedipus complex. It represents the young boy's fear that his father

▼ *A person with an inferiority complex may not trust friends to stick to arrangements.*

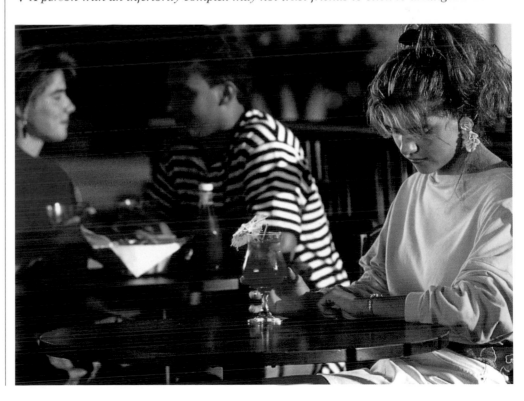

397

will cut off his genitals in revenge for his designs on his mother. However, there is a great difference between these ideas and reality. Very few boys show these tendencies or the behavior linked to them. Another well-known complex is the inferiority complex, a concept that was made popular by the psychiatrist Alfred Adler. Adler believed that the universal tendency in humans to succeed and to achieve is partly colored by the feelings of inferiority that are the inevitable result of the pressures of childhood. Small children are helpless; they have to do what their parents and other figures of authority tell them without argument and whether they like it or not. Very often they have to do what their elders tell them solely because their elders are bigger and stronger than they are, not because their elders are necessarily right. It is no wonder that many people have highly emotional ideas and memories of being inferior to those around them. For some people the memories persist into adult life. Two reactions can occur. The victims may take on an attitude of excessive humility and obedience to others, in an endeavor to escape criticism and the anxiety it produces. Or they may behave in a superior fashion, with an exaggerated sense of their own importance, so that no one can ever remind them of the inferiority they once felt and thus release the feared emotions.

Treatment

Not everyone acquires complexes, and some people grow out of them. But for those naturally anxious people who are prone to complexes, treatment is available. Complexes are learned; no evidence suggests that a person is born with them. This implies that any problem that an individual may have from such complexes can be solved, or minimized, by behavior therapy. Debilitating anxiety can be unlearned and a happier, more positive attitude adopted.

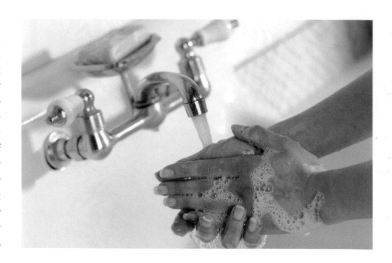

▲ *Constant, excessive hand washing is a common compulsion.*

Compulsions

A compulsion is an act that is carried out, usually repeatedly, to reduce anxiety. It may have developed from a pattern of behavior that was once normal. For example, a person may feel a compulsion to go around locking all the windows in his or her house. This is called obsessive-compulsive behavior (see Obsessive-Compulsive Disorder). Originally, it may have been a sensible precaution against burglars, but with the development of the compulsion the person feels the need to check over and over again that windows and outside doors, and even inside doors, cupboards, and boxes, are locked.

A compulsion may result from a superstition. An example of this is the game played by the fictional character Christopher Robin, who would never step on the cracks between sidewalk slabs because he believed bears were waiting around the corner to eat him if he did.

Almost everyone has minor compulsions that are hardly noticeable. People are creatures of habit, and a change can raise the level of anxiety. This is because it requires thought for a while, instead of automated programs of behavior. Small rituals are performed, such as tidying the pencil cup before leaving the office or plumping up the sofa cushions before going to bed. All are harmless ways of lowering arousal levels and relaxing, but excessive tidying, checking, hand washing, overeating, or avoidance of certain situations interfere with the smooth running of a person's life. The compulsion should be treated, and the anxious person may need support from a partner or a friend to get help.

One of the most effective methods of treating compulsions is a process called systematic desensitization. The patient learns to give him- or herself an instruction to relax, repeating a word such as "calm" until a tension-free state is achieved (see Tension). The situation producing the compulsive behavior is then called up, either in real life or in the imagination. When the compulsive behavior begins, the patient gives him- or herself the command "calm," and then senses his or her anxiety decreasing. As fear lessens, so does the need to behave compulsively. This boosts the patient's faith in the process. Soon the vicious circle is broken, and the obsessive behavior is eliminated or at least made manageable. Severe cases of compulsive behavior can be treated by cognitive behavior therapy.

See also: **Behavior therapy; Psychotherapy**

Some common complexes
Remember that the majority of complexes can be effectively treated by psychotherapy
Anxiety complex: excessive anxiety over an object or generally
Cain complex: strong rivalry between siblings
Castration complex: a son's fear of castration by his father
Electra complex: a daughter's wish to seduce her father
Inferiority complex: excessive feelings of inferiority leading to humility or its opposite, arrogance
Jocasta complex: excessive attachment of a mother to her son
Lear complex: excessive attachment of a father to his daughter
Oedipus complex: a son's wish to seduce his mother, which causes hatred of his father
Persecution complex: a belief that one is being victimized

Conception

Questions and Answers

We would like our next child to be a girl. Is it possible to influence the sex of our child during intercourse?

No. The sperm determines whether the child is female or male, and there is nothing a couple can do to make sure that either a sperm carrying a male chromosome or one carrying a female chromosome gets to the egg first. It has been suggested that the acid-alkali balance of a woman's vagina and cervical canal has some influence on sperm, and that an acid or alkali gel inserted into the vagina before intercourse may make it possible for the couple to choose a boy or a girl. There is no reason to suppose this method can work. Its reputation arises from the common fallacy of accepting evidence that supports the desired outcome and ignoring contrary evidence.

How long is the period during which conception is possible?

The egg lives for less than 24 hours after ovulation, which takes place in the middle of a woman's menstrual cycle; it is during this time that conception is possible. Sperm can live in a woman's body for 24–48 hours, or very rarely up to five days, so the egg may be fertilized by sperm as long as five days before ovulation.

My husband has a low sperm count. What can be done to help men with such a problem?

The sperm count is the number of sperm in 0.061 cu. in. (1 ml) of seminal fluid. Sperm cannot survive in high temperatures, so hot baths, tight underwear, or being overweight can cause a low sperm count. Too much alcohol or cigarette smoking are also likely to have a significant adverse effect on male fertility. If the low sperm count is caused by an inflammation or infection in the testicles, this can be treated by a doctor.

Knowing what happens during conception can help couples understand this complicated process and may help them overcome any problems they experience when trying to plan a family.

Conception is a great deal more complicated than the simple joining of a sperm and an egg. It is a complex process, and various conditions have to be right to ensure that it is successful.

Every time a man ejaculates, he produces sperm, but a woman is physically able to conceive only once during each menstrual cycle. Approximately 14 days before her period, she produces a single egg or occasionally two eggs from one of her two ovaries. The egg is then drawn into the fallopian tube. It lives for less than 24 hours, and if it is not fertilized, it dies and is absorbed into the cells lining the tube. The menstrual period follows 13 days later, and the cycle then begins again. The average cycle lasts 28 days, although some women find that their cycles are longer or shorter. Most women release approximately 12 eggs per year, if they have a regular 28-day cycle.

The sperm and ejaculation

If intercourse takes place around the time of ovulation, conception is likely (see Intercourse). A man produces about 400 million sperm in each ejaculation. These are surrounded by seminal fluid, which protects the sperm from the acidity of the vagina (see Semen). Once deposited, the sperm

HOW AN EGG IS FERTILIZED

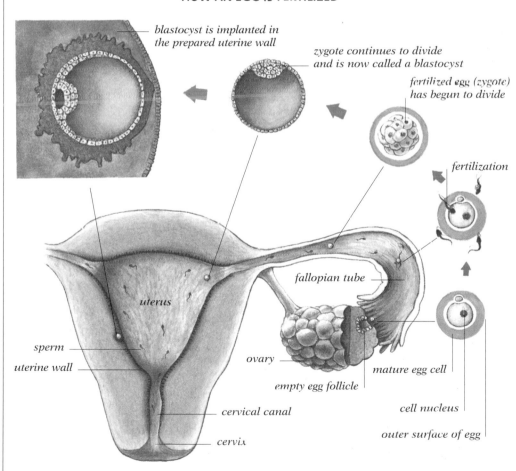

- blastocyst is implanted in the prepared uterine wall
- zygote continues to divide and is now called a blastocyst
- fertilized egg (zygote) has begun to divide
- fertilization
- fallopian tube
- uterus
- sperm
- uterine wall
- ovary
- empty egg follicle
- cervical canal
- cervix
- mature egg cell
- cell nucleus
- outer surface of egg

▲ An egg is released from one of the two ovaries, is fertilized by a sperm as it travels down the fallopian tube, and then implants itself in the wall of the uterus.

immediately start their journey up the vagina, through the cervix (neck of the womb), and into the uterus. They move by vigorously lashing their tails. Many of the sperm do not make this journey successfully and wither and die in the acidic conditions. This is nature's way of ensuring that damaged or unhealthy sperm do not fertilize the egg.

Fertilization

The millions of sperm that reach the uterus are nourished by the alkali mucus of the cervical canal. They then travel up into the fallopian tubes, a journey of about 8 inches (20 cm) that takes approximately 45 minutes. Only about 2,000 sperm may actually survive, but those that reach the fallopian tubes may stay alive within them for up to five days, ready to fuse with an egg if ovulation takes place. If an egg is already present within the tube, fertilization takes place immediately.

Fertilization occurs when a sperm penetrates the surface of the egg. Each sperm carries an enzyme (a substance responsible for activating biological chemical processes) that helps liquefy the outer surface of the egg to make penetration by a single sperm easier. Once the egg is fertilized, a membrane forms around the egg that prevents other sperm from entering. The egg and sperm (which has now discarded its tail) then fuse together to form a single nucleus (center), which then begins to divide into two cells. Within 72 hours, the cells divide five times to produce a 64-celled egg.

The fertilized egg travels down to the uterus in approximately seven days (day 21 of a 28-day cycle). During this time it grows tiny projections that help it burrow into the lining of the uterus, where it can be nurtured and a pregnancy can start (see Pregnancy). This process is called implantation; once it has occurred, conception is complete.

The egg can now be nourished by the rich blood supply present in the uterine lining. From the moment of fertilization, the egg produces a hormone called human chorionic gonadotropin (HCG), which informs the ovary that fertilization has taken place and maintains the blood flow to the lining of the uterus so that the egg can continue its development. (Pregnancy tests work by detecting this hormone in blood or urine.) The body therefore knows that the menstrual cycle must not continue, since a period would remove the fertilized egg.

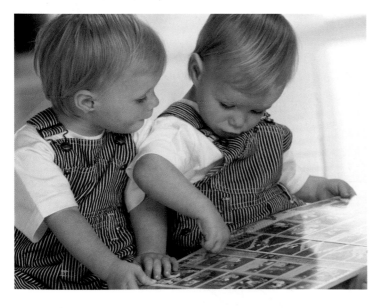

▲ *Identical twins are born when one egg is fertilized and splits into two as it begins to develop in the womb.*

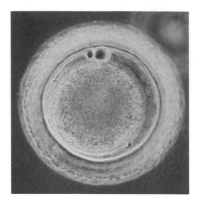

► *This photograph of a living egg, a few hours after fertilization, has been magnified 200 times.*

Not every conception occurs in this way. If the fertilized egg begins to divide and the two cells separate, they form two embryos, which become identical twins because they came from the same egg and sperm. Nonidentical twins occur when two separate eggs are released at ovulation and are fertilized by two separate sperm. Multiple births (three or more babies) occur for the same reasons, but although the use of fertility drugs has increased their number, they are still rare (see Multiple Birth).

Difficulties in conceiving

Although most couples conceive within six months, it can take up to two years for a woman to become pregnant. Even after two years some still find difficulty in conceiving. The cause of the problem may lie with either the man or the woman, or with both. The ease with which a woman becomes pregnant depends on her age and the age of her partner and the state of their health. Women are most fertile up until the age of 25; from 35 onward their chances of becoming pregnant decline rapidly until menopause. A man's decline in fertility is more gradual; at 60 he is still fertile, though to a lesser degree.

In spite of sex education, sexual intercourse for some couples may be unsatisfactory, although sex manuals and clinics may be helpful. Other couples have difficulties because they are unsure of the best time in the menstrual cycle to conceive; and when this uncertainty is combined with infrequent intercourse, the chances of conceiving are low. Emotional factors such as stress, anxiety, tiredness, or overwork can also play a large part in conception—intercourse may be less frequent, or the man may be incapable of maintaining an erection or of ejaculating during intercourse (see Erection and Ejaculation).

Women with infrequent periods ovulate less often, but they are still fertile, although their chances of conceiving may be reduced to only three or four times a year. A failure to ovulate, caused by thyroid problems, drastic weight loss, or premature menopause, is another common cause of infertility. There may also be a delay in the return of a woman's fertility after she comes off the Pill (see Oral Contraceptives). Damage to the fallopian tubes, arising from an infection in the tubes themselves (salpingitis) or other causes, will prevent them from functioning normally. Adhesions may form, which prevent the egg from passing down to the open end of the tube.

In men difficulties may arise when the testicles are not working properly, or there is a low sperm count. Diseases such as mumps may cause an inflammation of the testes, or there may be a testicle failure or a blockage in the vas deferens (down which the sperm travel) or epididymis (where sperm mature). There are many techniques to discover the cause of infertility and to help circumvent it.

See also: **Artificial methods of conception; Infertility; Menstruation; Ovaries; Sperm; Testes; Uterus; Vagina**

Congenital disorders

Many newborn babies have slight physical defects that are hardly noticeable or can be easily corrected. Serious defects cause great distress, however, so it is vital to take the preventive measures available.

Questions and Answers

I am going to be a grandmother soon, and although I don't want to scare my daughter-in-law, I would like to know if there are any blood tests for congenital diseases in newborn babies.

All babies have a blood test between the sixth and 14th days of life, called the Guthrie test, in which blood is taken by pricking the child's heel. The test detects a disorder of the body's chemistry called phenylketonuria, which can be treated with a special diet but would otherwise cause a mental handicap. As it occurs in only one in 12,000 babies, this is only a precaution. The test is also sometimes used to detect a lack of the thyroid hormone.

I am pregnant. Should I avoid taking any drugs or medicines in case they damage my baby?

Avoid taking any drugs during pregnancy. The most vulnerable time for the baby is in the first two months of pregnancy; you should particularly avoid taking any medicines then—not forgetting that conception occurs two weeks before you first miss your period. It is a good idea to stop taking any medicines if you think you might have conceived, even though many are perfectly safe. If you are taking a drug prescribed for a particular reason, consult your doctor, who will know if it could harm the embryo.

Someone told me that if I was frightened by an animal during pregnancy, the baby could be deformed. I am pregnant and have had dreams that my baby will be crippled. Is this possible?

There is no evidence that this can produce an abnormal baby. Many women have nightmares when pregnant—but if a woman who has had such dreams does have an abnormal baby, it is a coincidence.

Everyone hopes that a baby will be normal at birth, but some are born with an abnormality of some part of the body, or their internal chemistry does not work as it should. The word "congenital" simply means that the problem is present at birth; it does not mean the same thing as "inherited" or "genetic," although some of the problems do run in families (see Genetic Diseases and Disorders). Congenital disorders are still surprisingly common, occurring once in every 50 births, but many are relatively mild in nature and cause very little trouble.

Types

An example of a mild congenital disorder is the extra finger seen on some people, mainly from the West Indies. This defect passes from parent to child, and the extra finger is usually removed soon after birth. More serious disorders can often cause a baby's death shortly after it is born. This is particularly likely to happen with disorders of the heart and brain, which are relatively common (eight babies in 1,000 are born with congenital heart disease). Another medical riddle is the fact that some congenital disorders are regional, with a higher incidence in some parts of the world than others. Abnormalities of the brain and spinal cord were, until recently, found in one birth in every 2,000 in the United States; the most serious is anencephaly, in which the brain is exposed and incompletely developed. Spina bifida is a similar type of condition, in which the covering of the spine is not complete (see Spina Bifida). Unlike these defects, cleft lip and cleft palate are not as common in the the United States as in Japan and China (see Cleft Palate). Anencephaly and spina bifida are almost always avoidable now by having women take folic acid early in pregnancy.

Causes

In general there are two main groups of known causes: genetic or inherited problems, in which there was already an abnormality in the fertilized egg; and those where something has damaged the fetus in the womb during the earliest stage of its development (see Fetus). Some inherited problems, such as extra digits (fingers or toes), are actually seen in one of the parents as well as the child. In another type, each of the parents appears to be quite normal but has a gene that is passed on to the child, producing the problem. Cystic fibrosis (a serious malfunction of the glands) is an example of an inherited genetic problem (see Cystic Fibrosis). Both drugs and infections are

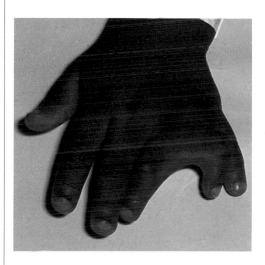 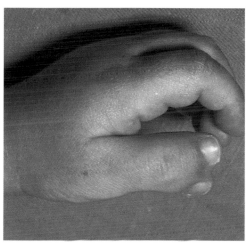

▲ *Webbed fingers (left), often accompanied by an extra finger or the presence of a double thumb (right), are fairly common deformities easily dealt with by surgery.*

known to damage the tiny, growing fetus. A tragic example of a manufactured drug that caused serious damage was thalidomide, which was originally prescribed to pregnant women to combat morning sickness, but which prevented proper growth of the baby's limbs and caused a whole range of other disorders (see Thalidomide).

German measles (rubella) can damage the heart, eyes, and brain of the fetus if the mother catches the disease—or has been exposed to it—during the first three months of her pregnancy; even after that time, it may cause deafness in an otherwise normal baby (see Rubella). Very often a combination of factors will lead to abnormality. Spina bifida is known to be the result of an embryonic problem called a neural tube defect. An adequate intake of folic acid from the start of pregnancy or before can prevent this (see Neural Tube Defect).

One special condition caused by the presence of an extra chromosome in each cell in the baby's body is known as Down syndrome. It is more common in babies born to older women, occurring once in every 1,000 babies born to 20-year-olds, with the occurrence rising to one in every 50 babies when the mother is over the age of 45. There are also many other chromosomal abnormalities.

Symptoms

In many cases the condition is obvious, but there may be internal problems resulting from the abnormality, as in spina bifida. Some internal conditions are recognized by their symptoms; a blocked gut, for instance, will cause vomiting within the first few days of birth and requires surgery. Breathlessness and a blue color to the skin, known as cyanosis, are often the result of heart conditions (see Blue Baby).

Sometimes a special test reveals the problem, as with dislocated hips. Since this condition is a recognized congenital disorder, every newborn baby is carefully examined to make sure his or her hips are normal and cannot be put out of joint (see Hip).

Treatment

The way a defect is treated very much depends on the nature and severity of the disorder. Some congenital disorders, such as the webs sometimes found between the second and third toes, need no attention. Others are relatively uncomplicated to deal with. Dislocated hips, if discovered early, can be treated with a splintlike support that is worn for a few weeks; if the condition is found later, an operation will be necessary. A blocked intestine or cleft palate can be dealt with fairly easily by corrective surgery. Abnormalities of the heart and brain are far more serious, though heart operations are becoming more successful. It is also possible to close the skin over the bare spinal cord of a baby with spina bifida, but a child born with an exposed brain cannot be helped. When an abnormality such as spina bifida arises, which can be improved with surgery, there is usually a discussion between the parents and the doctors to determine whether surgery should be carried out. It is not just a question of saving life, but also of considering the degree of physical and mental handicap the child will endure for the rest of his or her life.

Outlook

Some conditions improve with time, and some allow a normal life. For instance, the condition called hole-in-the-heart (ventricular septal defect) is really a muscular window between two heart chambers (see Heart). In the past this was thought to be permanent, but doctors now know that in more than three-quarters of cases, the hole closes by the time the child is eight years of age. Many children

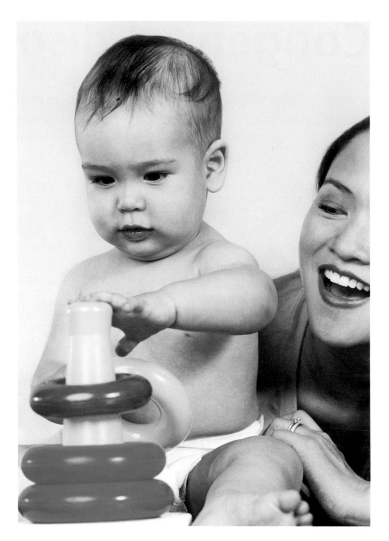

▲ *Many defects need no treatment; others, if caught early enough, can be helped by corrective surgery.*

can be helped by open-heart surgery, but many congenital disorders severely handicap the sufferer's life, so it is important that new ways should be found to prevent the abnormality from happening at all. When a couple know that there is an inherited illness in the family, they should consult a doctor, and possibly a genetic counselor, before planning to have a baby. Sometimes a test can be done during pregnancy that will detect an abnormality in the fetus, such as the test for Down syndrome, which is generally offered to all pregnant women over 40. To avoid the damage done by rubella, no woman should reach childbearing age without being protected by vaccination against the disease (see Vaccinations). In the case of spina bifida, there is some evidence that an improvement in the mother's diet can reduce the number of babies with this defect. This is an additional reason why balanced eating, with plenty of protein and vitamins—and not too many carbohydrates—should always be an important part of an expectant mother's prenatal program. If a child is born with a congenital disorder, physiotherapists, nurses, and health care workers, as well as the family doctor and specialists, can advise the family and help parents deal with problems that arise.

> *See also:* **Birth defects; Down syndrome; Pregnancy; Surgery**

Conjunctivitis

Questions and Answers

I have heard that contact lenses may cause conjunctivitis. Does this apply to both hard and soft lenses?

When contact lenses are first placed in the eye, they are like a foreign body, such as a speck of dust, and many people get an initial conjunctivitis. Usually it is not severe, but some people are particularly sensitive. Soft lenses cause less trouble, but there are advantages and disadvantages to both hard and soft lenses.

I have just had conjunctivitis. How can I avoid catching it again?

It depends on the type. Bacterial conjunctivitis will come back only if the source of the infection still exists: for example, if there is a sore elsewhere on the body. So the answer is to try to eliminate the infection. The cure for allergic conjunctivitis depends on finding the cause of the patient's allergy.

My young sister has conjunctivitis, and her eyes are sticky with pus when she wakes up. Will the rest of the family catch it?

The infection can be passed on if pus from an infected child gets onto someone's skin. You must make sure that nobody else uses anything that touches her face, such as a towel or washcloth.

My friend has had Bell's palsy and now has to wear special glasses to prevent conjunctivitis. Why?

Bell's palsy weakens or paralyzes the nerves controlling the muscles of one side of the face, including the muscle that keeps the eye tightly closed. The eye cannot shut properly, even during sleep, so it is easy for dust to blow into it, increasing the chances of getting conjunctivitis. Glasses can push up the lower lid to protect the lower cornea from drying.

Often known as pinkeye, conjunctivitis is a common complaint among young children and babies, who tend to rub their eyes constantly while playing. The inflammation usually responds quickly to treatment.

The thin, delicate membrane that covers the white of the eye and the underneath of the eyelids is known as the conjunctival membrane (or conjunctiva). Conjunctivitis is any inflammation of this sensitive membrane. The condition also causes inflammation of underlying blood vessels, which become large and pink as a result.

The type of conjunctivitis common among children is not serious, but there are other, more severe types, including one called trachoma—found mainly in Asia—that can ultimately cause blindness (see Blindness and Braille). Therefore, conjunctivitis needs to be seen by a doctor so that he or she can diagnose the type and determine whether it is infectious.

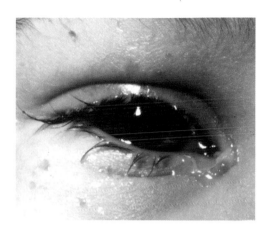

▲ *A child with conjunctivitis will often wake in the morning with pus or a watery discharge oozing from the infected eye.*

Causes and symptoms

Conjunctivitis is usually caused by viruses such as those that cause the common cold or cold sores, or a bacterial infection. Viruses are the smallest-known type of germ; bacteria are larger organisms that cause infection. The viruses are spread by droplet infection in the air breathed out by an infected person, or by contact with an infected object, such as a towel. The bacterial infections are usually caused by bacteria settling in the eye—perhaps from another infected area.

Other irritations or allergic reactions of the eye can also cause conjunctivitis—for example, if a speck of grit gets into the eye or if someone is suffering from hay fever. Such cases are not infectious. Too much strong light can have the same effect; and wind, dust, or smoke can also produce a temporary case of conjunctivitis. The condition may also be triggered by certain cosmetics, eyedrops, or contact lens solutions.

Symptoms and treatment

The common signs of the complaint are painful, red eyes; unusual irritation in strong light; and either pus or a watery discharge that makes the eyelids stick together first thing in the morning. In many cases the eyelids may swell up, too. Although the eye may itch, vision is quite normal.

Pus should be gently removed with salt water and clean cotton swabs; and if the condition is infectious conjunctivitis, the person's washcloth and towel must be kept separate to avoid passing on the infection. Antibacterial creams or drops, such as those containing chloramphenicol or neomycin, are frequently used to kill the bacteria or prevent damage from a virus, and antibiotics may be prescribed orally to clear up a recurring infection. If there is severe itching, the doctor may prescribe antihistamines. Dark glasses will also give some relief from discomfort.

Outlook

Most cases of conjunctivitis clear up completely within a few days. With trachoma, however, there may be damage to the eyelid and scarring of the cornea, and these defects will require corrective surgery (see Cornea). With allergic conjunctivitis, the cure may be more difficult, since the cause has to be identified and, if possible, removed. For this, the help of a doctor or possibly a specialist will be required.

See also: **Allergies; Antibiotics; Bacteria; Eyes and eyesight; Hay fever; Pus; Sty; Viruses**

Contact lenses

Many people prefer contact lenses to glasses because they feel that contact lenses improve their appearance. Observing high standards of hygiene and avoiding prolonged use are important if contact lenses are to be worn safely.

Questions and Answers

Can anyone wear contact lenses?

No. Some people simply cannot tolerate them—particularly the hard type—because of unusual sensitivity to discomfort. Other people have a medical condition that prevents them from wearing contact lenses—for example, those with allergies, hay fever, sties, or disorders such as excessive watering or bloodshot eyes.

If my daughter starts wearing contact lenses, will they stop her from becoming more nearsighted?

Unfortunately not. If her nearsightedness is hereditary and her eyesight is very poor, contact lenses will not prevent any further deterioration. If she does not like wearing glasses, however, contact lenses might be advisable for cosmetic purposes.

Can I sleep while wearing my contact lenses?

Most people remove their lenses at night for cleaning and reinsert them the following day. Napping while wearing lenses is common, but not everyone can tolerate this. Long-term-wear lenses are now condemned by ophthalmologists because of the high incidence of complications, some serious. Very thin soft lenses with a high water content may be worn quite safely for a day or two, but continuous wear is not recommended.

My soft lenses once caused abrasions on my eyes. Why did this happen?

Soft lenses require extra maintenance and a high standard of hygiene. Sometimes a film can build up on the surface, causing pain and swelling in the eye. Hold your lenses up to the light—if they appear cloudy or speckled, it is probably best to replace them.

A contact lens is a lens that fits over the front of the eye and is used in place of eyeglasses. Contact lenses are made of plastic and come in many colors.

Many people wear contact lenses for cosmetic or professional purposes, or for sports. They may also be worn for optical, medical, or surgical reasons.

Contact lenses can be used in cases where the iris has been lost through an accident or operation, because they can be custom-made to stop too much light from entering the eye. Similarly, cases of albinism—a rare condition in which the skin and hair are white and the irises red, making a person oversensitive to light—can also be aided by the use of special contact lenses.

Who can wear contact lenses?

People of any age can wear contact lenses, depending on individuals' state of health. They can be worn by people with myopia or nearsightedness, near-vision problems or hyperopia, corneal curvature anomalies or astigmatism, and even conical cornea or keratoconus, (see Eyes and Eyesight).

However, not all eyeglass wearers can actually tolerate contact lenses. They are unsuitable for people who have allergies, such as hay fever, which cause the eyes to run, or recurrent sties or other eye disorders, which the lenses might aggravate.

Choices available

Contact lenses are usually prescribed by an ophthalmologist (eye specialist) in either a hard or a soft variety. Hard lenses, made of an inflexible piece of plastic, are smaller, last longer, are less likely to cause infection, give excellent vision, and are less expensive than soft lenses. However, it takes longer to build up a tolerance to them.

Soft lenses, which are more pliable than hard lenses, are easily fitted to the eye. They can be tolerated more quickly and are infinitely more comfortable, even when first put in. However, the vision achieved is not as fine with soft lenses, and eye infections occur more frequently. Soft lenses are also likely to tear and do not last as long as hard lenses.

In the past, continuous-wear contact lenses were widely advertised and, for a time, seemed acceptable. More recently, experience has shown that problems are eventually likely to arise. In particular, wearing soft contact lenses for long periods can result in infection by an amoeba in the genus *Acanthamoeba*, which can cause serious corneal damage. There has been so much concern that some manufacturers are now offering "wear for a day and throw away" soft lenses.

Contact lenses can also be harmful if they cause abrasions of the tissues. Prolonged wear or wearing dirty lenses can lead to eye inflammations. Such complications occur rarely and are more common in the first two years.

Hard lenses, which are inserted into the eye with a lubricant wetting solution, must be cleaned daily. Soft lenses require a special nonirritant soaking solution.

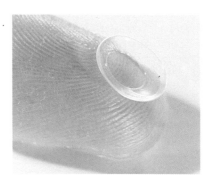

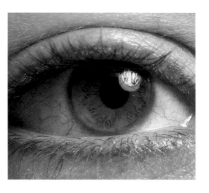

▲ *Before insertion, a hard contact lens is held on the fingertip (top). In the eye (above), it is hardly noticeable.*

See also: Allergies; Hay fever; Inflammation; Lazy eye; Ophthalmology; Sty

Contraction

If I have an IUD (intrauterine device) fitted, how long will it take to start working?

An IUD is effective as soon as it is in place. However, for the first three months, you must check the string once a week, because this is the time the IUD is most likely to be expelled. If that happened, you would no longer be protected.

I am 21 and would like to have an IUD fitted, but I've heard it is not suitable for women who have not had children. Is this true?

IUDs are not a first-choice method of contraception for women who have not had children, because the uterus and cervix have not been stretched by having a baby. This makes it more difficult and more painful to insert an IUD, and there is more chance that the uterus will expel it. There is also a higher chance of side effects such as painful periods, bleeding, and pelvic inflammatory disease (PID).

I am pregnant and want to have an IUD fitted after the baby is born. I plan to breast-feed my baby. Do I need to have it fitted during this time?

Some doctors like to fit an IUD soon after the baby is born; others prefer to wait six to eight weeks. Ask your doctor, and if he or she wants you to wait six weeks, you must use other contraceptive measures in the meantime. Just because you are breast-feeding does not mean that you will not get pregnant.

Can using a condom really keep you from catching sexually transmitted diseases?

A condom does give a high level of protection to both the man and the woman, but it cannot be relied on to give total protection.

Some contraceptives prevent pregnancy by creating a barrier between the sperm and egg; others either stop the fertilized egg from developing or convince the woman's body that it is already pregnant. Couples should think carefully and ask for advice about what method is best for them.

For thousands of years people have been trying different ideas to prevent women from getting pregnant, ranging from putting crocodile dung into the vagina to standing up after intercourse.

Nowadays the reproductive system is better understood, and more reliable methods are available. The Pill, an oral contraceptive, is one of the best-known, but not every woman can use it (see Oral Contraceptives). This article deals with the other effective contraceptive methods available.

Choosing a method of contraceptive can be confusing for a woman unless she knows how all of them work and what they do. Some methods are safer than others but may have side effects. Others are more difficult to use and have a higher failure rate. Some women are allergic to rubber and so are unable to use many forms of the diaphragm and condom. Others have heavy, painful periods, so an IUD (intrauterine device) would be unsuitable because it can accentuate menstrual pain and cause heavy bleeding (see Menstruation).

A woman should ask her doctor which methods are most suitable. If she goes to a birth control clinic, the clinic should be advised of her medical history. Whichever type of contraceptive she chooses, she should make sure she understands exactly how it works before using it.

In certain countries the use of contraceptives is barred or discouraged for religious reasons. In these places the only method condoned is the rhythm method.

Spermicides

Spermicides contain chemicals that kill sperm. They also inhibit the movement of sperm up the vagina and through the cervical canal (the passage into the uterus). Spermicides are not reliable on their own, so they are usually used with a condom or a diaphragm. Either of these creates a barrier between the man's sperm and the woman's egg (the ovum). If sperm somehow escape contact with the spermicide, the barrier will prevent them from reaching and fertilizing the egg.

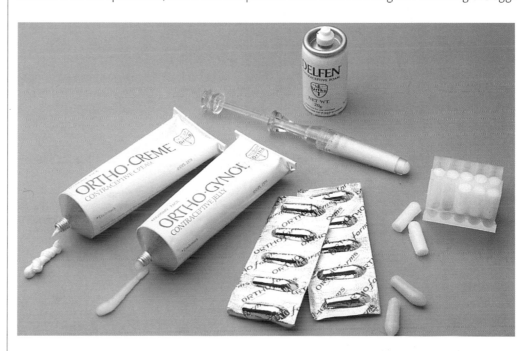

▲ *Spermicide, in the form of a cream, jelly, or pessary (vaginal suppository), should be used by the woman when she uses a diaphragm or when her partner uses a condom.*

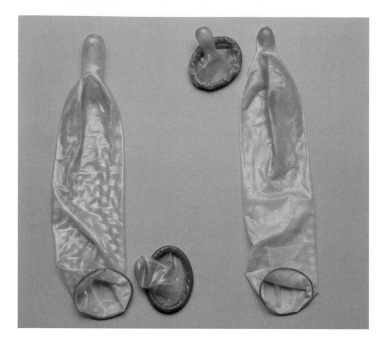

▲ *Condoms are tubes of fine rubber of varying thickness and texture that are unrolled to cover the erect penis.*

Spermicides are readily available from drugstores without a prescription and come in a variety of forms—pressure spray foams (which are the most reliable), tubes of cream and jelly, pessaries, and foaming tablets (which break up in the moist environment of the vagina and release chemicals). However, some spermicides have been found to be almost totally ineffective, and others can cause rubber to deteriorate. Before buying one it is wise to consult a birth control clinic to find out which brands are recommended.

The creams, foams, and jellies come with a syringelike applicator with a plunger. The woman fills the applicator with spermicide and puts it into her vagina, with the applicator tip as close to the cervix (the neck of the uterus) as possible to ensure that any sperm which get that far come into contact with the spermicide. The spermicide is released when she pushes the plunger down the applicator.

When to apply

Used with a diaphragm, spermicide can be applied up to an hour before intercourse. If a couple decides to use a spermicide on its own, they should apply it not more than 15 minutes before intercourse. However, this is not an effective method of contraception. If they have intercourse a second time, they should apply more spermicide, as there is enough in one application to deal with sperm from only one ejaculation. The woman should not wash away the spermicide sooner than six to eight hours after intercourse.

Pessaries or tablets should be put in place only two to five minutes before intercourse, because they are not effective for very long. The woman can use her finger to place the pessaries as high up in the vagina as possible.

Condoms

Known by a variety of names—including French letter, sheath, rubber, protective, and prophylactic—a condom is a tube of fine rubber that is closed at one end. In its package, it is rolled up so that it looks like a flat circle with a thick rim. It unrolls as it is pulled over the erect penis. It can then catch all the semen that the penis ejaculates and stop it from reaching the uterus (see Semen). In addition to being a method of contraception, condoms are also recommended as a barrier against AIDS (see Sexually Transmitted Diseases).

The tip of the condom should be held between the forefinger and thumb of one hand while it is put on, because this keeps air out and allows some space for the ejaculatory fluid. This method also reduces the risk that the condom will burst.

The condom should be put on not only before the penis enters the vagina but before it even touches the woman's genitals. This is because semen can leak out of the penis throughout foreplay. One complaint about condoms is that the couple must stop foreplay to put the condom on. However, many couples overcome this problem by making it part of their foreplay.

There are lubricated condoms available; the lubrication prevents the condom from tearing when it enters the vagina. If this type is not being used, it is a good idea to use spermicide as a lubricant (petroleum jelly should not be used, as it destroys rubber). It is better to use a spermicide in any case, as an extra precaution, since it is always possible that a condom is faulty. When the penis is withdrawn from the vagina, either partner should hold the condom at the base of the penis so that the penis does not slip out and allow semen to escape.

Condoms are available in many countries in a choice of textures, sizes, and colors, without prescription, from drugstores and mail-order companies. They are the only method of contraception, apart from a vasectomy (surgery that permanently prevents the presence of sperm in the ejaculation), in which the man takes total responsibility. Condoms are 96 to 97 percent effective when used properly with a reliable spermicide.

The female condom is made of plastic and is less likely to burst than a conventional male condom. It offers excellent protection against both conception and infection, since it covers the whole of the vulva and vagina. However, it is not popular with many couples.

Diaphragms

A diaphragm is a round, dome-shaped contraceptive made of rubber or plastic. It is inserted into the vagina and covers the cervix, preventing any sperm from entering the uterus (see Cervix and Cervical Smears). There are three different types of diaphragms, but they all work on the same principle. Used correctly—with spermicide—they are 96 to 97 percent reliable.

The Dutch diaphragm is the largest type, varying from 2 to 4 inches (5 to 10 cm) across. It has a strong spring in the rim, and when it is in position, the front of the rim rests on a little ledge on the pubic bone and the back in a small crevice behind the neck of the uterus. Dutch diaphragms are the easiest to use and for this reason are the most popular. But they are not suitable for women who have poor pelvic tone, because these women's muscles are not strong enough to hold the diaphragm in place. Such women should be able to use another type of diaphragm.

The cervical diaphragm is much smaller than the Dutch diaphragm and looks like a thimble with a thickened rim. Some women find it more difficult to handle and insert, and men can sometimes feel it during intercourse because it is not as flat as the Dutch diaphragm.

Finally, the vault diaphragm is a cross between the previous two types. Unlike the others, it can be made of plastic, so women who are allergic to rubber can use it. Like the cervical diaphragm, the vault diaphragm can occasionally be felt by the man.

HOW TO INSERT A DIAPHRAGM

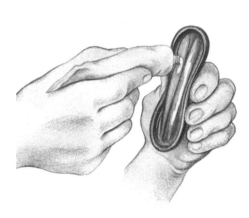
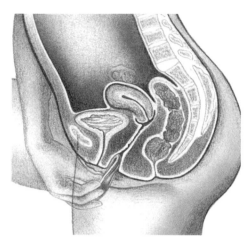
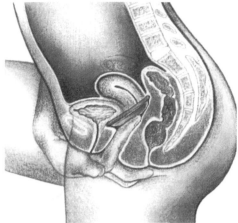

▲ *Place spermicide on both sides of the diaphragm and smear more around the rim. Squeeze into a cigar shape with the fingers.*

▲ *Squat or raise one leg, and after spreading the lips of the vagina, push the diaphragm deep into the vagina until it is in place.*

▲ *Be sure that you can feel the cervix through the diaphragm. Leave the diaphragm in place for at least six hours after the last ejaculation.*

Using a diaphragm

It is not possible to go to a drugstore and buy a diaphragm. A nurse or doctor must fit it to make sure it is the right size, as every woman is slightly different. A properly fitted diaphragm should stay in place during intercourse without causing discomfort to either the woman or her partner. If it is uncomfortable or if it moves, then either it has not been fitted correctly or it is not the right type of diaphragm for the woman concerned.

The couple should always use spermicide with a diaphragm, as a second line of defense, just in case any sperm get past. A spoonful of spermicidal jelly or cream should be squeezed onto both sides. Then more jelly or cream should be smeared all around the rim. To insert the diaphragm, the woman squeezes it into a cigar shape using the thumb and finger. She then uses one hand to spread the lips of the vagina while the other inserts the diaphragm. It is usually easier to insert if she squats down, as this shortens the length of the vagina.

The woman can check the position of her diaphragm by making sure she can feel the cervix through it. The doctor will show her how to do this when the diaphragm is fitted. If intercourse does not take place until more than an hour after insertion, she should apply more spermicide without removing the diaphragm. The woman should leave the diaphragm in place for at least six hours after intercourse, since sperm can live this long in the vagina. To remove a Dutch or vault diaphragm, hook a finger over the rim and pull. Cervical diaphragms have a string that can be pulled to remove them.

The woman should wash the diaphragm thoroughly in warm water after use and check it for any small holes, especially around the rim. If there is a fault, she should replace the diaphragm, using an alternative contraceptive method in the meantime. The diaphragm should be dried thoroughly and stored in the container provided, away from direct sunlight.

▶ *All varieties of diaphragm—cervical (top left), Dutch (right), and vault (bottom left)—are used with spermicide. If necessary, this can be reapplied with a special applicator (bottom right) when the diaphragm is in place.*

A diaphragm should be checked by the doctor at least once a year to make sure that it still fits correctly and does not need replacing. This annual check is especially important if the woman has recently had a baby, has gained or lost an excessive amount of weight, or has only just started to have an active sex life (see Sex).

Benefits

The most important benefit of the diaphragm is that it has virtually no side effects. Occasionally it may cause a slight vaginal irritation, and some women find that it brings on cystitis (inflammation of the bladder). These conditions are relatively minor, and after diagnosis

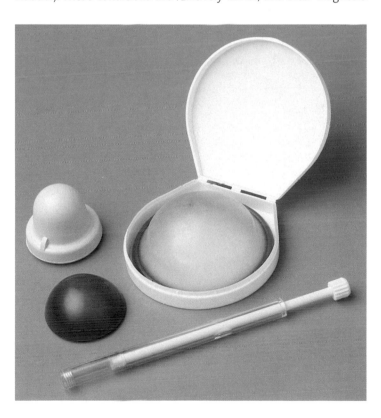

Questions and Answers

I have heard that there is a condom available which covers only the tip of the penis. Would this kind increase sensation for the man during intercourse?

This type of condom is often referred to as an American tip. However, it is not reliable as a means of contraception, even if used with spermicide, because it can easily slip off.

I like the idea of having a Dutch diaphragm because it has no side effects. But isn't it a messy method of contraception?

It all depends on how squeamish you are—some women do not like to use tampons, for instance. A diaphragm does involve using spermicide, so it is messier than an IUD. It also takes a conscious effort to use. On the other hand, there are fewer side effects. You really need to weigh the advantages and disadvantages.

I have just been fitted with a Dutch diaphragm, but the clinic said I must use a spermicide with it. I do not see why, provided the diaphragm is a good fit.

Even though the diaphragm is fitted for your size and has a strong spring to make sure it stays in place, sperm are tiny and there is always the possibility that they could swim around the edge of the diaphragm and into the uterus. However, if you use spermicide around the rim of the diaphragm and on the side nearest the uterus, it will kill any sperm that do get past.

Can I use a diaphragm during my period?

Yes. All that happens is that the diaphragm holds back the menstrual flow until it is removed. Keep it in for six hours after intercourse, and then use a pad or tampon as usual. Intercourse during a period can be less messy, and therefore more pleasant, if you do use a diaphragm.

by the doctor they can be treated easily and effectively. Nonetheless, a few women find that they cannot use any type of diaphragm. This may be because their muscles are too relaxed for it to stay in place. In addition, some young women may have a vaginal opening that is relatively small, and they have difficulty inserting a diaphragm. Other women find it too distasteful to use. Not all contraceptives are suitable for every woman. Doctors will help each woman to find one that is right for her.

Intrauterine devices

Intrauterine devices—commonly known as IUDs—work in a different way from condoms and diaphragms. They are inserted into the

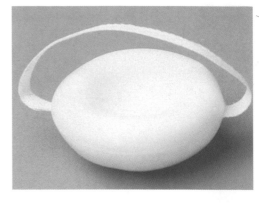

▲ *The vaginal sponge works a little like a diaphragm. The loop aids removal.*

uterus and, rather than forming a barrier between the sperm and the egg, they prevent a fertilized egg from implanting in the uterus. Doctors are not sure exactly why IUDs work, but they are known to prevent the lining of the uterus from thickening—so the right environment for an egg to develop is not created. An IUD does not require any preparation before intercourse. The reliability rate of IUDs is 98 percent, slightly higher than that for diaphragms and condoms.

Internationally, and over the years, IUDs have been made in many shapes and sizes. There are two types currently available in the United States: the ParaGard Copper T 380A, which contains copper and can be left in place for 10 years; and the Progestasert. The Progestasert is a hormone-releasing IUD that is thought by doctors to be more effective than earlier IUDs and less likely to cause excessive bleeding (see Hormones). There is, however, still a risk of ectopic pregnancy (in which the fertilized egg lodges in the fallopian tube). Unlike the ParaGard Copper T 380A, the Progestasert IUD must be replaced every year.

Insertion

Most IUDs are supplied to the doctor or clinic in sterilized packs with a fine plastic tube, about 0.08 inch (2 mm) in diameter, for insertion. An IUD is usually implanted during or just after menstruation, because the cervix is more relaxed at this time. The depth of the uterus is checked by passing a small probe through the neck of the cervix. This shows the doctor how deep to insert the IUD. The IUD is straightened out inside the tube, and the tube is inserted through the cervix. When the correct depth is reached, the tube is detached and the IUD springs back into shape inside the uterus. The whole process is simple and takes only a few minutes.

The insertion may be a little painful for some women, especially if they are nervous and tighten up their muscles. If there is any pain, however slight, after more than a few days, the woman should go back to see her doctor.

Disadvantages

Some women may find that they have heavier periods than usual for the first two or three months after having an IUD fitted, and sometimes there may be slight spotting between periods, backache, or stomach cramps. These symptoms usually disappear after a couple of months, but anyone who is having a lot of pain should see her doctor.

Occasionally an IUD may be expelled from the body for no apparent reason other than that the woman's internal anatomy was unsuitable. If this does happen, it is usually within the first three months and can be during menstruation, when it may pass unnoticed. All IUDs have a fine nylon string attached that hangs down into the vagina, and it should be possible to feel this with a finger. If the string cannot be felt, or if it seems longer than usual, the woman should consult her doctor. She should use another method of contraception in the meantime.

After having an IUD fitted, the woman should check the string once a week for the first three months. After this she should check it once a month after menstruation, as this is the time the IUD is most likely to become dislodged. Some men complain that they can feel the string during intercourse. If this bothers them, a doctor can shorten the string. Tampons rarely get caught up in the string, but if the woman feels a sharp pain when she removes a tampon, she should check the string. Some types of IUD can be left in place for several years, but the woman should have

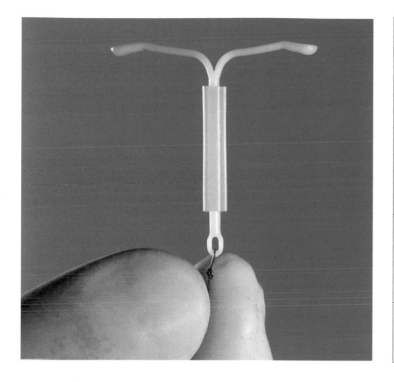

▲ *One of two IUDs currently used in the United States, the Progestasert is a hormone-releasing device. As with all IUDs, the fine plastic string at the bottom hangs through the cervix into the vagina, making removal easy.*

The rhythm method

The rhythm method of contraception relies on the fact that a woman is fertile for only a few days in each menstrual cycle. By determining which days these are, she can avoid pregnancy by avoiding intercourse on her fertile days.

The two or three days just after ovulation are the fertile days, so to avoid conception, no intercourse should take place during these days. Because sperm may live for 24 to 48 hours in the female reproductive tract, it is also wise to avoid intercourse for the few days before ovulation.

In order to determine when she will ovulate, a woman needs to become aware of, and to monitor, her temperature, the condition of the lower part of the uterus, and the production of fertile mucus (which keeps the sperm alive and guides them to the entrance of the uterus).

Although the rhythm method is better than using no contraception at all, it is not very reliable, and really should be used only if no other alternatives are possible.

a medical checkup at least once a year. A woman is unlikely to get pregnant with an IUD in place, but if she suspects she has conceived, she should see her doctor at once (see Conception). The IUD must be removed, because it could cause a miscarriage.

Morning-after IUD
If a woman has had intercourse at the midpoint of her cycle—her most fertile time—without using any contraceptives, some doctors will fit an IUD afterward. This must be done within 72 hours of intercourse. It can be removed at the next menstruation. A better alternative may be the morning-after pill (postcoital contraception), although some people's religious beliefs prevent them using either of these methods as they may be considered a form of abortion.

Douching
It used to be thought that semen could be flushed out of the vagina with hot water or a mild solution that is hostile to sperm. Women used to insert a syringe with a rubber bulb at one end into the vagina and then squeeze out the contents. However, not only is this method totally unreliable, but it can also be dangerous—a dirty syringe can cause an infection (see Sex; Sperm).

Vaginal sponge
Usually made from polyurethane foam, the vaginal sponge fits over the cervix in the same way as a diaphragm. It is impregnated with spermicide that is released gradually over a 24-hour period. The sponge works in three ways: it blocks the entrance to the uterus, thereby preventing sperm from entering; it absorbs sperm; and the spermicide kills sperm on contact. The sponge must be left in place for at least six hours after ejaculation.

New methods
The following are some of the new methods of contraception that are now available to women.

Depo-Provera shot: This is an injection of the female hormone progesterone, which is given about every three months. It works by inhibiting ovulation, and by preventing sperm from reaching the egg and the fertilized egg from implanting in the uterus. It is as reliable as the Pill (which is 99 percent-plus reliable), but because it does not contain estrogen, many of the dangers and side effects of the Pill are absent (see Estrogen). It is especially good for women who have difficulty in remembering to take the Pill on a regular basis.

Lunelle shot: This is an injection of the hormones progesterone and estrogen, which is given about once a month. It is as reliable as Depo-Provera; its side effects and dangers are similar to those of the Pill.

NuvaRing contraceptive ring: This is a flexible ring about 2 inches (50 mm) in diameter that is impregnated with progesterone and estrogen and fits inside the vagina in the same way that a diaphragm does. It releases the hormones into the body in the quantities normally present during pregnancy, fooling the body into thinking it is pregnant so it does not release any eggs. The woman wears the ring for 21 days, then removes it to allow menstruation. After seven days she inserts a new ring, and the process is repeated. It is 99 percent reliable.

Ortho Evra patch: This is a skin patch about 1 3/4 square inches (18 mm²) worn on the buttocks, lower abdomen, or upper body, which releases estrogen and progesterone into the bloodstream. The woman replaces the patch with a new one once a week for three weeks, then removes it for a week to allow menstruation. The skin patch is 99 percent reliable, although it seems to be less effective for women who weigh more than 198 pounds (90 kg).

See also: **Abortion; Abstinence; AIDS; Cystitis; Ectopic pregnancy; Erection and ejaculation; Genitals; Hysterectomy; Intercourse; Pelvic inflammatory disease; Penis and disorders; Uterus; Vagina; Vasectomy**

Convalescence

A patient's attitude, together with care and attention from their family, friends, and health workers, all contribute to a speedy recovery. This is particularly the case after surgery or a serious illness.

Anyone who has spent a few days sick in bed will know the feelings of weakness and fatigue that accompany the early days of recovery (see Fatigue). These sensations are even more extreme in people who have had a serious illness or operation.

Discharge from the hospital depends not only on the speed and degree of recovery but also on the kind of care available afterward. Older people living alone are usually not discharged until arrangements have been made for help and care at their home.

Caring for any convalescent can be an enormous strain, and caregivers often take on more than they can cope with rather than face the possibility of feeling guilty or disloyal. As a result they risk stress for themselves as well as for the patient (see Stress). It is far better to be realistic about taking on caring tasks and to ask for any necessary help at an early stage.

A few hospitals offer special rehabilitation programs: patients return on an outpatient basis to learn, for example, how to walk after a stroke, or to how to adjust to arthritis. Relatives are sometimes invited to take part so that they know what type of help to offer the patient.

Diet and supplements

The modern approach is not to give convalescing patients a special diet, except perhaps for the first few days after an operation or when a specific diet is necessary. A normal diet should consist of light, nourishing meals with plenty of fruit and vegetables, milk, cheese, eggs, meat, and fish. The doctor may suggest extra vitamins. If he or she does not, a general multivitamin supplement from a drugstore will do no harm—though the doctor's advice should be sought.

Often a patient suffers a dramatic drop in weight after an illness; this causes more weakness. If his or her appetite is poor, small meals at shorter intervals may be more inviting.

Exercise and activity

In the hospital it is common to see postoperative patients tentatively making their way around the ward as part of their exercise routine. At home, daily activity is a good idea in most cases, along with any specific exercises advised by the hospital. There may be instructions to avoid lifting heavy objects or engaging in active sports, but otherwise patients are usually allowed to set their own pace.

Postoperative depression

Early recovery often seems fast and dramatic, particularly if the patient has been in intense pain. Sudden relief from this can seem miraculous, and there may be an unrealistic surge of optimism. But depression due to fatigue may follow, and if this persists for any length of time, it may need treatment (see Depression).

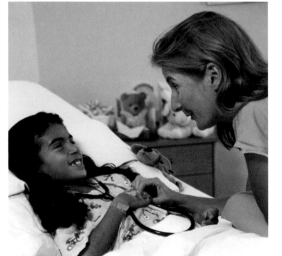

▲ *Family and friends can make all the difference to a young patient.*

> *See also:* **Appetite; Arthritis; Diet; Exercise; Home care; Mind-body therapy; Nutrition; Outpatients; Physical therapy; Postoperative care; Rehabilitation; Stroke; Weight**

Questions and Answers

My mother has always believed in taking a good tonic after an illness. Is there any value in this?

The idea of a tonic has gone out of fashion, although tonics may still be prescribed, perhaps more as a psychological boost than for any medical value. Most commercial tonics contain vitamins and minerals or are simply glucose drinks that are easily digested to give instant energy. They are not strictly necessary but do no harm. A nourishing diet is the best tonic.

Why do doctors give a patient sleeping pills after an operation?

Sleep aids recovery, and discomfort may cause a person not to sleep well after surgery. For this reason a short course of sleeping pills may be advised by the doctor. A good diet can help sleep. A painkiller in conjunction with a sedative is a good idea, but a hot, milky drink at bedtime also makes good sense.

In the past, I used to read about people being sent to the seaside for convalescence. Is sea air really good for you?

The idea that a visit to the seaside provides beneficial effects in convalescence is now known to be a myth. The only good thing about sea air is that it is less likely to be polluted and is therefore good for those with lung complaints.

My friend can afford to stay at a health spa regularly, and it makes her feel really fit. Is this a good idea after an illness?

It depends on the spa. Make sure that the place is well-established, that there is medical supervision, and that it is geared to the convalescent's needs. A short vacation in a pleasant climate may be equally beneficial.

Convulsions

Questions and Answers

My brother goes to a lot of clubs. Can convulsions be brought on by the flickering lights?

Yes. Many people cannot tolerate the strobe lights in clubs, since the frequency of the flicker induces a type of temporary short circuit in their brains. This causes the brain to assume a particular frequency of brain wave, which brings on a seizure. However, if your brother is susceptible, he will have been affected by now.

My toddler has temper tantrums. Could these bring on convulsions?

Convulsions can be triggered by a severe temper tantrum. Breath-holding is a sign of this—the child appears to be holding his or her breath deliberately, inducing unconsciousness and convulsions. Despite appearances, they are rarely serious, and you must just wait for the symptoms to abate.

I suffer from convulsions. Is it safe for me to drive?

There is the possibility of a seizure while driving; also the side effects of some drugs slow reactions.
  For these reasons, people who need drugs to control convulsions should neither drive nor operate hazardous machinery. Two seizure-free years without medication generally indicate an adequately controlled case, but laws concerning driving vary from state to state.

Is it true that some foods and drugs can bring on convulsions?

Allergies to certain foods may bring on a form of convulsion, although such reactions are rare. Convulsions may also be a symptom of food poisoning. Certain drugs may cause convulsions if given in improper doses or to susceptible patients.

Convulsions can have a number of causes, including epilepsy, a reaction to a high fever, and poisoning. Remaining with the patient, staying calm, and performing simple first aid can do a lot to help.

The most common cause of convulsions in infants and young children is a fever or sudden rise in temperature. This type of convulsion is known as a febrile convulsion, and it is unlikely to occur after age five. During a febrile convulsion the head and body will jerk, the eyes will roll, and the child may hold his or her breath. The legs and arms may stiffen and the back arches. The treatment is to lower the child's temperature by sponging him or her with tepid water, and to protect the child from injury by placing rolled towels around him or her. The child must not be cooled too much and as soon as his or her temperature is normal (98.6°F/37°C), cooling should be stopped.

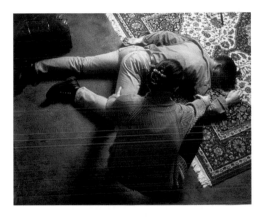

▲ *Stay with a person until the seizure stops, then place him or her in the recovery position and get help.*

Epileptic seizures

An epileptic seizure is a major electrical disturbance in the brain that results in loss of control and muscle spasms. The person becomes unconscious and falls down. He or she may twitch uncontrollably and writhe and shake. The eyes roll upward, breathing becomes labored, and there is sometimes frothing at the mouth. His or her teeth may be clenched violently, and if the tongue is in the way, it may be badly bitten. Spontaneous emptying of the bladder or bowels may also occur. Such convulsions last only a few minutes, and afterward the sufferer falls asleep, perhaps after briefly recovering consciousness. Epileptic seizures can affect either specific parts of the body or both consciousness and muscle function. If a person has an epileptic seizure, he or she should not be left alone to call for help—the attack will last for only a short while. Bystanders should ensure that the victim's head is protected and that tight clothing around the neck is loosened. Once the convulsion is finished, the victim should be placed in the recovery position (see Epilepsy).

Other types of convulsions

In a newborn baby, convulsions may be caused by brain damage or central nervous system disorders; epilepsy is a likely cause. Convulsions can also arise from occupational hazards such as poisoning from lead or mercury. Very low blood sugar levels can trigger a convulsion caused by an imbalance between insulin and food intake. People who drink heavily over a long period or who are trying to give up drinking alcohol are also prone to convulsions.

Dangers and first aid

In addition to the possibility of biting the tongue, injury can result from falling onto a hard object or striking furniture while writhing on the floor. If possible, place a small pad, such as a folded handkerchief, between the victim's teeth. If the teeth are clamped shut, they should not be forced open, and fingers should be kept out of the person's mouth. Serious complications and possibly death can result if the person vomits and chokes, or inhales vomit into the lungs. If there is vomiting, the head must be turned to one side so that the person does not choke. If a convulsion occurs when a person is driving or using machinery, the consequences could be fatal. When he or she comes to or falls asleep, call a doctor immediately.

> *See also:* **Breath holding; Fevers; Food poisoning; Nervous system; Poisoning; Temperature; Unconsciousness**

Coordination

Questions and Answers

My son has suddenly become very clumsy. Will he grow out of this?

A child's lack of coordination can happen for various reasons. At different stages of growing up, such as at the start of puberty, children may seem more clumsy because they are not concentrating as well; any emotional upset will have the same effect. However, if the clumsiness has occurred out of the blue, it would be worthwhile to consult your doctor.

My uncle has recently lost an eye. Will this affect his coordination?

Probably not. Each of the two visual centers in the brain receives information from both eyes, so the loss of one eye does not affect someone as badly as the loss of one field of vision (that is, the left or right half of each eye's sight). The brain can also compensate for the loss of vision in one eye. However, if the visual centers are damaged through a stroke, and half of the visual field is lost, then a person will have difficulty in judging distances, particularly gaps such as doorways, thus appearing to be clumsy or lacking in coordination.

I know a man who always staggers around as if he were drunk. Could this be because of an ear disease?

The inner ear has mechanisms that provide information about the position of the head, which is essential for equilibrium and balance. In old age these often become defective, but in younger people disease of the inner ear rarely occurs. Disease may cause symptoms such as unsteadiness of the limbs or vertigo (a spinning sensation), since the brain is receiving the wrong signals about the orientation of the head. A similar effect occurs when a person is spun around rapidly for several seconds.

Why do some people seem to be natural athletes, dancers, or gymnasts, while others seem to be less gifted? The answer lies in the complicated processes of coordination that begin in the brain.

The supple movements of a champion gymnast reveal, in their flowing patterns, how delicately the human brain can control the hundreds of muscles in the torso and limbs. To achieve such intricate sequences of action, the human brain has evolved a complex system of control and guidance that makes even the most sophisticated computers look primitive.

Babies are born with many reflexes (muscular responses that occur without conscious thought). To visualize these reflex actions in an adult, imagine how quickly a person would withdraw his or her hand from a hot saucepan. The movements that are directed by the brain (voluntary movements) are superimposed onto these simple reflex actions. For every action that is performed, some muscles contract, others relax, and still more maintain their contraction to stabilize the rest of the body. The process by which all the individual muscle contractions are carefully synchronized to produce a smooth order of activity is called coordination.

How coordination works

To understand this process, consider an everyday action such as leaning over a table to pick up a cup of coffee. How does the brain direct this apparently simple task? Before someone can pick up a cup of coffee, a series of events must happen.

First the person must know where the cup and his or her hand are and the relationship between them. This means that the brain must be able to generate a "map" of the space for necessary movement to be planned. This is called spatial perception. The brain must then interpret this internal "map" of the outside world so that the problem of getting the coffee cup from the table to the hand can be solved. It must then generate a plan of action that can be translated into a detailed set of instructions to the muscles so that they will contract in the right order.

During the movement, started by the planning parts of the brain (the premotor area), continuous streams of information pour in from all the sensors (nerves) in the muscles and joints. This information, which has to be organized and relayed back to the brain, describes the positions of the muscles and joints as well as their states of contraction.

In order to move the hand to pick up the cup of coffee, the person also needs to lean slightly toward it, and this alters the center of gravity of the body (see Balance). All the reflex balance mechanisms must be controlled to ensure that the correct changes in muscle tone are made, allowing the movement across the table that the brain has ordered. This means that the background tone of many other muscles has to be monitored and coordinated.

First stages of coordination

All intentional movements need to be practiced before they become coordinated. Even such ordinary actions as walking are

▲ *A game such as golf requires a great deal of coordination between the hands and eyes.*

HOW THE BRAIN ENABLES US TO PICK UP A CUP OF COFFEE

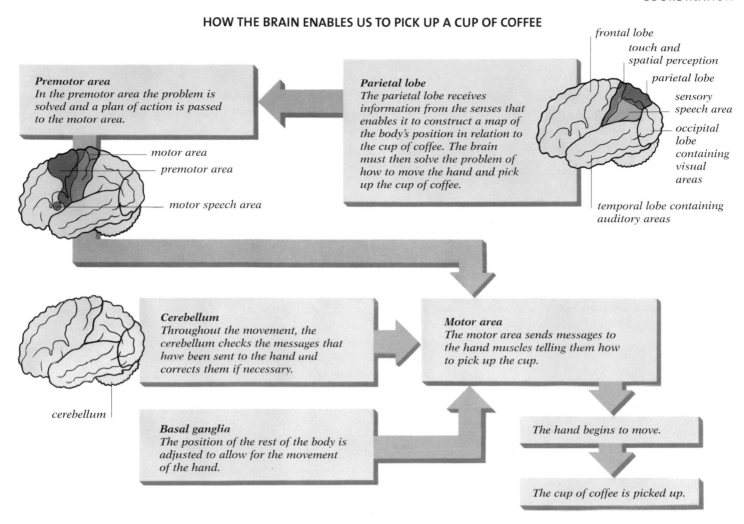

Premotor area
In the premotor area the problem is solved and a plan of action is passed to the motor area.

motor area
premotor area
motor speech area

Parietal lobe
The parietal lobe receives information from the senses that enables it to construct a map of the body's position in relation to the cup of coffee. The brain must then solve the problem of how to move the hand and pick up the cup of coffee.

frontal lobe
touch and spatial perception
parietal lobe
sensory
speech area
occipital lobe containing visual areas
temporal lobe containing auditory areas

Cerebellum
Throughout the movement, the cerebellum checks the messages that have been sent to the hand and corrects them if necessary.

cerebellum

Basal ganglia
The position of the rest of the body is adjusted to allow for the movement of the hand.

Motor area
The motor area sends messages to the hand muscles telling them how to pick up the cup.

The hand begins to move.

The cup of coffee is picked up.

major problems for every developing child. As a baby's brain matures and the interconnections increase, the primitive reflexes with which he or she was born (such as the startle reaction, which causes the hands to be outstretched when a baby feels he or she is falling) are overlaid with progressively more complicated ways of moving.

A toy might attract the baby's eye, because its bright color causes a strong signal in the visual centers, but the baby finds that reaching out is not enough to touch this object, so he or she is impelled to move toward it. The first attempts to move are not coordinated: the limbs just thrash around. But these initial attempts enable the necessary brain connections to develop for the set of actions that make up a coordinated crawl. Once crawling has been achieved, the messages sent from the brain to the muscles can be improved on until nothing at ground level is safe from the child's grasp.

When the baby discovers that he or she can get into an upright position, the cerebellum (the part of the brain responsible for coordinating voluntary muscular activity) has to analyze new instructions coming from the balance centers in the brain stem. Walking is another new skill to learn, requiring many attempts during which the cerebellum cooperates with the motor area to develop efficient messages to send to the muscles.

The separate parts of each action learned in this way are preprogrammed into the spinal cord, but they must form a coherent pattern to produce a coordinated movement, in the same way that an orchestra must have a conductor before it can produce a tuneful sound from all its instruments. Once these "simple" skills have been perfected, the brain has been programmed so that no concentration is necessary—the premotor area says "walk," and the right set of instructions go into action to produce the complicated mechanical actions that are involved. The cerebellum monitors the progress of the action, but this is less and less a conscious event. If a "problem" is introduced into the system, such as the change in the foot's posture caused by wearing high heels, some reprogramming is necessary, and concentration is needed while the motor cortex learns this new "tune."

Advanced coordination

In complex movements, the movement of the eyes is coordinated with the visual receptive centers of the brain and then with the movement of the rest of the body. This coordination is the last to mature. It forms the basis for learning the type of complex movements that are needed in sports or in skills such as playing a musical instrument.

Some brains seem better equipped from birth to develop in particular ways. However, to a large extent, abilities in complex types of coordination depend on how much the individual can concentrate to build up these specialized "programs" for complex movements.

See also: **Brain; Movement; Muscles; Reflexes**

Cornea

Is having an eye graft painful?

The procedure, lasting about half an hour, is performed under a local or general anesthetic. The eye may feel a little bruised, but there is seldom more than mild discomfort, and usually the patient is too happy with the result to notice any soreness. If sutures (stitches) have to be removed, a short stay in hospital may be required, but a buried continuous suture is often left.

Will my eye look different in shape or color if I have an eye graft?

If the eye needing the graft is scarred, a white area will show up on the cornea. After a successful graft, your eye will look much more normal, since the operation will bring back the color of the iris. The scar from the operation is visible only at very close range.

Can I become a cornea donor?

Anyone can become a donor, as long as the eyes are free from disease or injury. Contact your nearest eye hospital, and tell your doctor and your nearest relatives.

How can I take care of my eyes to keep them functioning well?

Ideally, let nature do the work. Tears contain a natural antiseptic, which eye baths can wash away. Do not use drops or put anything in your eye unless a doctor prescribes it. If you get grit in your eye, wash it out with a mild salt and water solution.

Is it true that a disease of the cornea can cause blindness?

A chlamydial infection, trachoma, is still common in underdeveloped countries, and it can cause blindness even in children.

The cornea—the eye's main lens—is the shining, transparent bulge at the front of the eye. If it is scarred or damaged, sight is impaired, but a graft operation from a donor eye can sometimes be performed to improve vision.

The cornea, together with the fluid behind it, forms the powerful, fixed-focus lens of the eye. It measures just 0.02 inch (0.5 mm) thick at the center and 0.04 inch (1 mm) thick where it joins the white of the eye, the sclera. The optical power of the cornea accounts for about two-thirds of the total eye power.

The cornea consists of five layers. On the outside is a five-cell layer called the epithelium, which corresponds to the surface skin. Underneath this is an elastic, fiberlike layer called Bowman's layer. Next comes the tough stromal layer, made up of a protein called collagen. The stromal layer is the thickest part and contains various infection-fighting antigens that help keep the cornea free from infection. It is also thought to help control inflammation in the cornea.

After the stroma comes a layer called the endothelium, which is only one cell thick. This layer keeps the cornea transparent and maintains a balance of water flow from the eye to the cornea. Once formed, the cells of this layer cannot regenerate, so injury or disease to the endothelium can cause permanent damage to sight. The final layer, called Descemet's membrane, is an elastic one.

A tear film covers the epithelium. Without tears the cornea would have no protection against bacterial microorganisms, pollution, or dust. The tear film is also essential for vision, since without tears the epithelium would lose its transparency and become opaque.

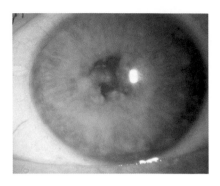

▲ *This diseased cornea has lost its transparent quality, affecting the focus of the eye.*

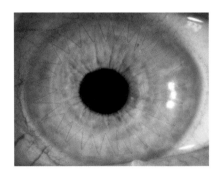

▲ *The same eye five weeks later. Note the fine zigzag line holding the clear grafted cornea in place.*

Corneal grafting

This operation is done on diseased or injured corneas when the central portion is scarred or the curvature is deformed. Where the cornea is deformed, the irregular surface causes gross distortion of the image on the retina, and very poor vision (see Blindness and Braille).

A disk is cut out of the cornea, removing the diseased area or scar tissue. Most grafts done to restore sight are around 0.27 inch (7.5 mm) in diameter. There are two procedures: one is to cut the full thickness of the cornea, the other is to cut only part of the thickness. The latter operation, called a lamellar graft, is usually done to replace diseased surface tissues, when the deeper tissues are still in good shape. The donor eye has a similar-size disk cut from it, and this is placed in position over the living eye and sewn into place using an operation microscope and fine nylon or collagen thread mounted on a curved needle 0.16 inch (4 mm) long.

In most instances the patient is allowed to leave the hospital within a few days, and many notice an improvement in their sight even in this short time. If the graft starts to be rejected, anti-inflammatory drugs are used, and in many cases the graft survives. Stitches may be removed several months later, and then, provided that the graft is clear, the sight is corrected by glasses or contact lenses. At this point, if the operation has gone well, the patient should notice a great improvement in his or her sight. The graft will leave only a faint scar.

See also: Eyes and eyesight; Grafting; Scars

Corns

Corns are localized areas of hard, horny skin formed by repeated rubbing or pressure. They are so common that most people have had them at some time in their lives. Corns can usually be treated at home or, if severe, by a podiatrist.

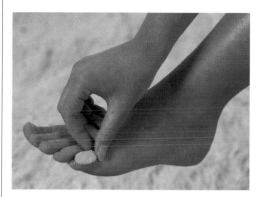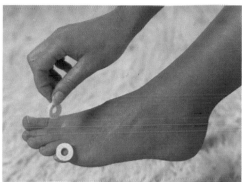

▲ *Corn plasters (left) contain an acid that softens the hard skin so that it can be removed more easily. Corn pads (right) can be used to protect corns from rubbing.*

Corns are hardened areas of skin that form as a result of repeated rubbing or pressure. Dead skin cells build up and create a thickening of the keratin (protein) in the skin, which inflames the deeper skin cells underneath, causing pain and discomfort. Very large corns are usually called calluses.

Causes

Corns are likely to occur whenever and wherever there is excessive wear on the skin. Manual laborers and people who go barefoot develop pads of hard skin that are quite normal, never painful, and, therefore, not true corns. In other people, such as violinists (who are continually rubbing their chins against wood) and anyone wearing a new pair of tight shoes, pads of skin may form at the site of the rubbing, causing considerable pain. These are true corns.

Badly fitting shoes and high heels tend to cause corns. The most common sites are on the ball of the foot, the sides of the toes between the joints, and sometimes the heel.

Corns frequently form over bunions, although there is no special association between the two. The reason is simply that the bunion, being a swelling on a prominent bone, presses against the inside of footwear, causing pressure. Corns invariably appear over bony prominences, where the hard skin protects delicate structures underneath. Some people are more susceptible to corns than others; this is particularly true of the elderly.

Calluses can also develop where artificial limbs or appliances rub on the skin. They are a normal response to excessive wear. In some cases they can be useful, because they take the brunt of pressure and impact and protect the skin; but occasionally they may become uncomfortable and need trimming.

Symptoms

A corn can be recognized as an area of hard, thick skin that often looks yellow compared to the surrounding skin. It is often conical in shape. Corns between the toes can be soft.

SECTION THROUGH A CORN

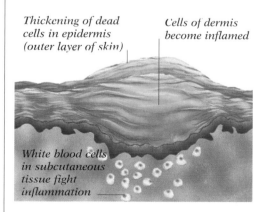

Thickening of dead cells in epidermis (outer layer of skin)

Cells of dermis become inflamed

White blood cells in subcutaneous tissue fight inflammation

▲ *A corn is an area of hard, thickened skin, beneath which the skin cells have become inflamed.*

Causes and treatment of corns

TYPE OF CORN	CAUSE	TREATMENT
Simple corn (on ball of foot, on side of toes between joints, on heel)	Excessive pressure on the skin. Occurs primarily because of tight shoes, but corns can also appear where there is a wearing away of the skin over a bone.	**Remedial action** Wear soft, good-fitting shoes with pads or arch supports on areas likely to rub. **Self-treatment** Small corns: Soak in warm water, and rub pumice stone over corn. Well developed corns: Gently pare off skin with a clean scraper or corn-paring knife. Or apply a corn plaster containing a chemical softener directly over corn; leave for 24 hours; lift off corn with pumice stone or corn-paring knife. Or pad corn with a ring of foam rubber surrounding the corn. **Treatment by a podiatrist** People suffering from persistent corns, or those who have arthritis or who suffer from diabetes or circulatory disorders, should consult a podiatrist.
Calluses	Same as above, but calluses are larger and can arise when artificial limbs or appliances rub on the skin.	Same as above. The best remedy for calluses is to alleviate the cause of the rubbing or pressure.
Corn on bunion	Bone of bunion pressing against the side of footwear.	Same as above. The best form of treatment is to have the bunion removed surgically.

Corns may first be noticed because they cause aching at the end of the day or because they feel tender under pressure. When corns are chronic or severe, the surrounding area may be slightly red, and the corns may be extremely painful, even when the patient is at rest. Symptoms vary considerably, and it can be difficult to tell a corn from a wart on the sole of the foot. In general, plantar warts are initially small and painful under pressure. When the top skin is rubbed off, tiny black roots will appear as dots; the area may then look like a wart.

Dangers

Corns are uncomfortable and painful but rarely dangerous. The chief danger is that, as the skin is pared off as part of treatment, infection may occur owing to the use of unclean instruments, so corns should be pared very carefully. This is particularly important for corns on the foot of a diabetic, who is likely to have poor circulation and in whom any infection can easily turn gangrenous. Treatment is best undertaken by a qualified podiatrist (chiropodist or foot specialist).

Treatment

Because corns are made up merely of hard skin, they can usually be treated by removing the excess skin. After a good soaking in the bathtub, rub a pumice stone over the corn. This is enough to keep some people's corns at bay. For more well-developed corns, scraping off the skin with a scraper or paring the corn with a safety knife is often necessary. The tools used should be kept scrupulously clean. The fine slivers of dead skin should be removed until soft, pliable skin is felt beneath the corn. Care should be taken not to pare away too much

skin: this could cause bleeding or introduce infection. Other tools that can be used to remove corns include a clean file and an emery board.

Corn plasters remove the skin by softening it with chemicals: a 40 percent salicylic acid solution is soaked onto a plaster, which should then be applied directly over the corn and left for 24 hours. The skin should then be lifted off with a pumice stone or corn grater. If the corn persists, further applications of plasters may be used.

Some older people become so accustomed to tolerating a corn that they stop taking care of it, simply padding it to ease the pain. Various products are available for this purpose, the simplest being a ring of foam rubber on a sticky base with a hole in the middle. Calluses can also be treated by applying a special solution containing salicylic acid on a plaster and then paring down the callus. Diabetics and those with circulatory disorders should have regular professional podiatry (chiropody) to ward off infection (see Gangrene).

Outlook

An isolated corn that has occurred because of a change of footwear or activity can usually be treated easily and should not recur. Calluses tend to need regular, permanent attention and will disappear only if the cause is removed. Recurrent corns over the bones of the foot or between the toes will need regular, professional treatment. Wearing correct footwear can help, but such corns tend to be chronic.

Pain and aching from a corn should never be accepted: corns can usually be treated, although they do tend to recur.

See also: **Bunions; Feet; Podiatry**

Coronary arteries and thrombosis

Questions and Answers

Could I have had a minor heart attack without knowing it?

Yes. It is fairly common to find clear evidence of a previous heart attack on the electrocardiogram of a patient who has never had any symptoms. These so-called silent heart attacks are most common in the elderly.

How old do I have to be before I am at risk of a heart attack?

Heart attacks are occurring in younger and younger patients. They occasionally occur in the teens and twenties, but they are more likely from the late thirties and early forties onward.

Does jogging lessen the risk of coronary disease?

Exercise requiring stamina gives some protection, and jogging, cycling, swimming, or walking are good for you. Muscle- or body-building exercises are unlikely to give protection unless they are part of a controlled gymnastic program. If you have been sedentary all your life, do not suddenly start exercising; build up gradually.

Why is my angina much worse in cold weather?

If you exercise in the cold, the circulation in the skin shuts down and increases resistance to the blood flow and heart action. Exercise only when warmed up.

My doctor says not to take the beta-blocker drugs for angina because I am asthmatic. Why?

Asthmatics should not use them because they cause wheezing and breathlessness.

What happens when people experience a coronary thrombosis, or a heart attack? And what are their chances of leading an active life again? Advances in medicine can do much to help, but prevention is better than treatment.

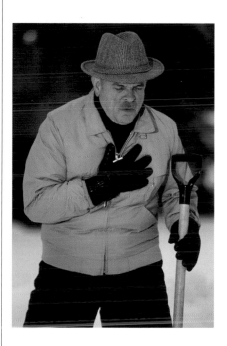

▲ *A heart attack causes severe, crushing pain in the chest.*

The coronary arteries are the vessels that supply blood to the heart itself. They are particularly prone to partial or total obstruction by atheroma—a buildup of fat that is caused by many factors, but principally by excessive stress, sedentary living, smoking, and an unhealthy diet. Obstructed coronary arteries are the cause of heart attacks; disease of the coronary arteries is the most common cause of death in the majority of Western countries.

The three arteries

The heart is a muscular bag that pumps blood around the body. Like any muscle, it has to be supplied with oxygen and food to continue working. This supply is carried in the right and left coronary arteries, which are the first vessels to leave the aorta (the body's main artery) as it emerges from the heart. Almost as soon as it branches off the aorta, the left coronary artery splits into two big branches. So there are, in effect, three coronary arteries: the right plus the two branches of the left. They go on to completely surround and penetrate the heart, supplying blood to every part of it. The coronary arteries are particularly affected by any obstruction because, like the heart itself, they are always in motion and the resulting strain on their walls hastens the buildup of atheroma. Atheroma is the principal feature of the arterial disease atherosclerosis. Except in a tiny proportion of cases, the disease process is always the same. Fatty deposits build up on the wall of the artery, narrowing the whole artery and creating the risk of a total blockage.

Heart attack

If a coronary artery becomes completely blocked, the blood supply to an area of heart muscle is shut off. There is an intense, heavy pain, often lasting for hours or even days, and described by the patient as resembling a viselike grip. The patient also experiences shortness of breath, cold sweat, and palpitations of the heart, and he or she looks very pale. Eighty-five percent of those who have a heart attack recover, but in some patients there is another, sometimes disastrous, attack in the first hour. After the attack, the area of heart that was affected eventually heals into a scar. That particular part of the heart muscle will never work again. But with careful treatment the patient will, in most cases, be able to lead a healthy, active life once more.

The blockage itself usually comes about as a result of what is known as a thrombosis (blood clot). The artery, narrowed by atheroma, restricts the flow of blood to such a slow pace that its natural tendency to clot or thicken begins to operate. This clot makes the final obstruction. A heart attack is often referred to as a coronary thrombosis, or simply a coronary (see Thrombosis).

The other problem caused by coronary artery atherosclerosis is angina. In this case there is a partial block that allows the heart to function normally during rest but does not allow the extra blood flow necessary for exercise. In some patients the pain of angina is caused by intense

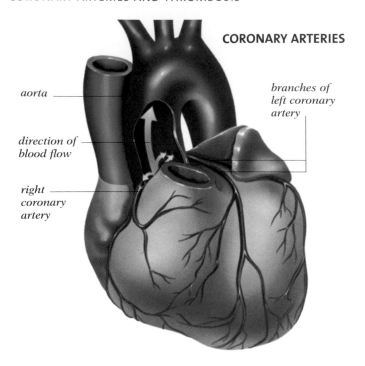

CORONARY ARTERIES

aorta

direction of
blood flow

right
coronary
artery

branches of
left coronary
artery

◄ *Three main coronary arteries supply the heart muscle with oxygen and nutrients: the two branches of the left coronary artery, and the right coronary artery.*

Treatment

Angina can be a crippling disease, even when the patient has not suffered a heart attack. At his or her worst, the patient may not be able to move more than a few yards without pain. Fortunately modern drug treatments are now available that temporarily widen the coronary arteries.

Patients can carry these drugs with them. When slipped under the tongue or taken by inhaler, they quickly stop attacks; but they are not very good at preventing an attack, because their effect lasts only for a few minutes.

Beta-blockers, however, have been a more lasting treatment for angina since their development in the mid-1960s, a great medical advance. These drugs block some of the effects (the so-called beta effects) of adrenaline. In doing so they also reduce the amount of work the heart has to do and, therefore, its need for oxygen. Taken regularly, not just when there is pain, they reduce the number of angina attacks and help prevent heart attacks.

For people who cannot take beta-blockers because they suffer from asthma, there is an alternative treatment with calcium channel blockers, which interfere with the movement of calcium through cells to help reduce the workload on the heart.

Surgery

There have recently been considerable advances in surgery for the treatment of coronary artery disease. In bypass grafting, the surgeon removes a length of vein from the leg and uses it to connect the diseased blood vessel directly to the aorta so that blood bypasses the

spasm of the coronary arteries rather than actual physical blockage. This type of pain manifests itself at rest rather than during periods of exercise.

This relative lack of blood flow produces pain. The typical angina chest pain spreads to the arms, shoulders, or neck. It is usually brought on by exertion or excitement and lasts only a few minutes. Patients who have angina may develop a full-blown heart attack, and, conversely, patients who have had a heart attack may get attacks of angina.

Symptoms of heart attack and angina

	HEART ATTACK	ANGINA
Type of pain	Dull, crushing, or heavy pain, "a tight band around the chest." Patient often describes the pain by clenching a fist. A sure sign is that nitrate drugs will not relieve the pain, as they do the pain of angina.	May be heavy or dull pain, or may be sharp.
How long the pain lasts	More than half an hour, often much longer.	Minutes only.
What brings it on	May come on at rest or during sleep, but may be precipitated by exertion, excitement, or a heavy meal.	Almost always brought on by exertion or excitement, but also by sudden exposure to extreme cold.
What stops it	Usually nothing.	Stopping the exertion; glyceryl trinitrate or trinitrin under the tongue.
Sweating	Usual.	Rare.
Nausea or vomiting	Usual.	Rare.
Breathlessness	Common.	Uncommon.
Patient's appearance	Often very sick-looking with grayish skin.	Most patients know they have angina and may not give any signs of pain or distress.

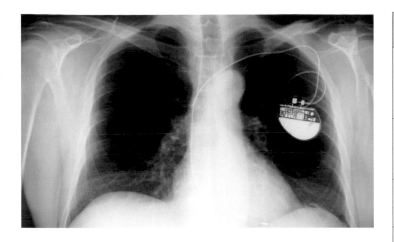

▲ *If the heart's timing system is severely impaired, a pacemaker can be implanted in the chest that sends out an electrical impulse to make the heart beat at the correct pace.*

Coronary disease—Who is at risk?

Smoking 10 cigarettes a day doubles the chances of a coronary, since nicotine in the bloodstream causes the arteries to go into spasm, narrowing them and making thrombosis more likely.

People who are more than 20 or 30 percent above the usual weight for their age, height, and sex are two to three times more prone to heart disease than people of average weight.

Anyone who has been under work or family pressures for a long time is at definite risk of a coronary.

People in desk jobs who do not exercise are certainly more at risk than active people.

People who eat large amounts of cholesterol in dairy foods or animal fat are at risk and should adjust their diet.

People from families in which there is a history of heart disease should be sure to exercise and eat a healthy diet.

obstruction. Successful bypass grafting depends on sophisticated surgical techniques. The joins must be able to withstand high pressures, and the blood vessels are only a few hundredths of an inch (a few millimeters) wide. There is no doubt that such surgery can be effective at relieving angina pain. It is also possible to attach an artery from the chest wall to the blocked artery.

Another important procedure to relieve angina is angioplasty. This is done using a special tube called a balloon catheter. The catheter is passed along the coronary artery until the tip, bearing the balloon segment, lies in the narrowed section. The balloon is then inflated with fluid under pressure so that the atheromatous plaque is compressed into the wall and the vessel widened. The results of balloon angioplasty are usually excellent.

Treatment problems

The reason why blood flow in coronary arteries becomes obstructed is still being extensively investigated. But one fact seems clear: blockage nearly always occurs when there is atheroma. Death from heart attacks occurs for two basic reasons. First, the death of an

Preventing coronary disease

Exercise regularly: swimming, walking, and jogging are ideal, although people who have been sedentary for a long time should avoid suddenly starting vigorous exercise. Build up gradually, and if in doubt, ask the doctor's advice. When exercising, think about the exercise, not personal or work problems. If work involves sitting at a desk all day, walk as much as possible instead of driving; take the stairs, not the elevator; and seek medical advice about an exercise program that can be done while sitting.

Eat a sensible diet: cut down on potentially harmful substances such as animal fats. Replace butter with certain types of margarine and use sunflower or canola oil for cooking. Cut down on sugar and starch, and avoid large, heavy meals.

Reduce mental stress: stress is part of living, but the body is not designed to put up with it constantly—so slow down!

area of heart muscle, caused by the blocked artery, causes a major disturbance of heart rhythm, which reduces the efficiency of the heart so severely that it may stop working. Second, if too much heart muscle is destroyed, the heart is simply not powerful enough to pump an adequate amount of blood around the body. In contrast, relatively minor disturbances of heart rhythm—known as arrhythmias—can usually be treated with drugs or by giving electrical shocks. If the timing sequence becomes totally interrupted, however, and the heart slows or even stops—a condition known as a heart block—it may be necessary to use a pacing system.

Pacemaker

A wire is passed into a vein and threaded in the direction of the blood flow, until it becomes lodged against the wall of the heart. The other end of the wire is connected to a pacemaker implanted in the chest. This sends out a regular electric impulse that drives the heart at the correct speed (see Pacemaker).

Recovery

After one or two days in a coronary care unit, heart attack patients usually spend about 10 days to two weeks in the hospital. During this time they gradually regain their strength and resume normal activities as much as possible.

After leaving the hospital and returning home for a period of recuperation, most people are well enough to go back to work within two or three months of a heart attack. In general, patients are encouraged to resume an active and normal life. There is no need for anyone to overprotect the heart or to consider the patient a permanent invalid. In fact, a lack of exercise or activity may probably have been a major cause of the heart attack in the first place.

See also: Calcium; Electrocardiogram; Exercise; Heart; Heart attack; Heart disease; Pain; Surgery

Cosmetics

Questions and Answers

My 13-year-old daughter is already using creams on her face. Will this be damaging to her skin?

Your daughter's skin is unlikely to be so dry that it needs a cream to soften it, and it will benefit from a moisturizer only when exposed to extreme weather conditions. If she uses a cream that is too heavy or applies it incorrectly, she may damage the tissue. This could cause wrinkles as she gets older.

I've started making my own beauty preparations, but they do not last. What am I doing wrong?

Homemade beauty preparations, though often very effective, do not contain the preservatives found in manufactured cosmetics. You should make only small quantities at a time, and store them in the refrigerator.

My mother is in her forties, and her skin is very dry and developing a lot of lines. What is the best treatment for this?

She should protect and lubricate her skin day and night with a rich moisturizing cream. This will make the lines less noticeable, although it will not slow down the rate at which they appear. She should use a rich cleanser, followed by a diluted toner. The most important thing is to avoid exposure to strong sunlight.

I cannot afford expensive creams, but I do want to take care of my skin. What do you suggest?

Ignore advertisements for miracle skin creams, and do not be impressed by fancy chemical terms that seem to promise wonders. Healthy skin does not need expensive creams. If you have a skin problem, speak to your doctor or pharmacist. There are plenty of inexpensive creams on the market.

Skillfully used, makeup can disguise defects, such as scars and birthmarks, and will also enhance a person's best features. Although rarely harmful in themselves, however, cosmetics should be applied with care.

Modern cosmetics are generally problem-free, thanks to strict controls on ingredients, labeling, and safety. Correctly applied, cosmetics can have a dramatic effect on the way a person looks and feels. Cleansers and moisturizers also form a large part of the cosmetics market.

Cleansing and deep cleansing

Cleansing is the most important treatment for the skin. Some people like to use cleansing lotions or creams, while others prefer plain soap and water. As long as people use a gentle complexion soap, soap and water does not harm the skin. Makeup, however, must be removed with a cleanser. The face should not be cleansed more than twice a day.

Many products are specially formulated to have a chemical affinity with the skin. When the face is cleansed with soap, it can take hours to return to its natural, slightly acidic state. However, using a pH- or acid-balanced product will help the skin remain in this state even while being cleansed. Some cleansing products are medicated, but they should be used only with a doctor's advice, because their antibacterial agents can irritate.

One of the best cosmetics for cleansing deep down in the pores is the face pack or mask. Made of a sticky substance such as clay, rubber, or wax, it is applied to the skin, then either rinsed or peeled off. The fresh, glowing look that masks produce is only temporary, but they do clean out clogged-up pores. All face packs should be kept clear of the delicate eye area.

Toning the skin

All cleansing lotions and creams tend to leave a filmy residue on the skin. If a person uses these to cleanse, he or she will have to use a toning lotion afterward to remove the residue. Toner will also "plump up" the skin cells, although, again, the effect is only temporary.

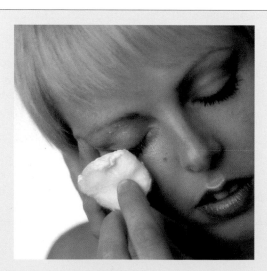

1. Eye makeup should always be removed at night. A special eye makeup remover is best because it is designed to shift the most stubborn makeup, yet still treats this delicate area gently. Always use quick, light movements.

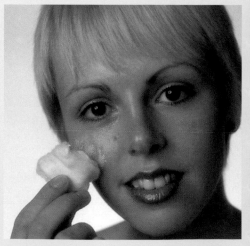

2. The rest of your makeup should also be removed, or pores may become blocked, leading to acne or infection. Use either a makeup remover followed by facial soap and water, or a lotion or cream that cleanses and removes makeup. Use the same movements as for applying moisturizer (step 4).

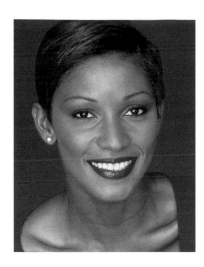

▲ *When skillfully applied, makeup can disguise problem areas and enhance a person's best features.*

Toners are perfectly safe provided that the one used is of a strength appropriate to a person's skin type. Toners known as fresheners are the mildest, and they are suitable for dry skin, whereas astringents contain the most alcohol and are suitable only for oily skin.

Moisture barrier

There is also a vast range of moisturizers on the market, from the lightest lotions to the heaviest night creams. Their main contribution is to help seal in the skin's moisture. Oily skin needs less help with this, since its oil content provides a natural seal against moisture loss. However, as a person grows older, the skin becomes drier and less efficient at keeping moisture in. This is when moisturizers become useful.

Some moisturizers are sold on the basis that they keep the skin looking young by attracting moisture from the atmosphere (see Aging). Others contain supposedly rejuvenating ingredients, such as collagen (a protein substance that makes up the underlayer of skin) and vitamin E. Despite these claims, there is little evidence to indicate that such additives have any substantial effect on the skin. Many women believe that the more moisturizer they apply, the more they are keeping wrinkles at bay. But wrinkles begin deep down in the skin and using more than a thin film of moisturizer can actually damage this layer. The key to preventing wrinkles lies in avoiding long exposure to intense sunlight and using protection if exposure is unavoidable. People should also be careful when using cleansers and moisturizers—applying them too vigorously or with downward movements may strain facial muscles and result in extra lines (see Wrinkles).

Using makeup

While makeup does not actually do the skin any good, most of it does not do any harm either. There is no denying the psychological boost that makeup can give. Skillfully used, it can minimize or hide problems and highlight good features. Foundations and cover sticks cover red veins, pimples, and under-eye shadows and can even improve skin tones. Green powder will tone down very red coloring.

Most skin troubles are caused by poor hygiene. Keep brushes very clean, and do not lend makeup to other people. Never spit on eye shadow or lick eye pencils—this can lead to infection (see Hygiene).

Caring for the eyes

Eyeliner worn on the rim of the lower lid often leads to infection, as does failure to remove eye makeup, especially mascara, each night, because the hair follicles become clogged. Always use quick, gentle movements when applying or removing makeup around the eye area. This tissue is delicate, and it is easy to create extra wrinkles. If redness, itching, or swelling occurs, an allergy to one of the dyes, scents, or other ingredients is possible. Try using a different brand or hypoallergenic cosmetics, which do not contain the ingredients that commonly cause allergic reactions.

> *See also:* Acne and pimples; Allergies; Bacteria; Birthmarks; Cosmetic surgery; Infection and Infectious diseases; Scars; Skin and skin diseases; Sty; Sunburn; Veins; Vitamin E

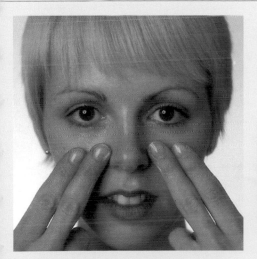

3. If you have cleansed with a lotion or cream, you will need to follow this by using a toning lotion. This gives skin a tingly, fresh feeling and removes the residue left by the cleanser. Toner can also be used after soap and water but is not strictly necessary.

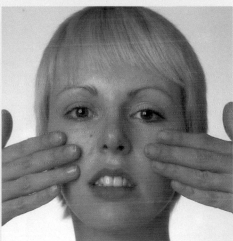

4. If you have dry skin, you should apply moisturizer morning and night. Use gentle, upward movements. Massage the cream in quickly, starting at the chin and moving up across the cheeks to the ears, then from the nose to the temples and across the forehead. Treat the eye area very gently.

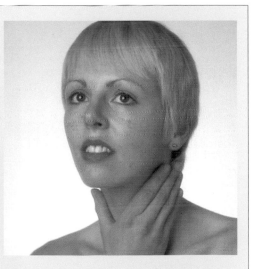

5. Do not forget to moisturize your neck and throat, too, using long strokes from the collarbone up to the jaw. In addition to being exposed to the elements, this area has a natural tendency to dry up. If neglected, the neck and throat will be one of the first areas to show signs of age.

Cosmetic surgery

Sometimes perfectly healthy individuals choose to undergo cosmetic surgery to make their appearance more attractive. All operations carry a risk—a person should think very carefully before making this decision.

Cosmetic surgery is a branch of plastic surgery that is carried out to change the shape of the body or to reconstruct or repair soft tissue. Cosmetic operations can have psychological benefits, improving the patient's self-esteem. They may also have some medical benefit.

Cases for treatment

A badly shaped nose, or one that is too big or too small, can be improved with rhinoplasty (a "nose job"). This involves reshaping the nasal bone and sometimes the cartilage (the stiff tissue at the end of the nose). Rhinoplasty is often done for cosmetic reasons, but also to correct breathing problems caused by a broken nose or misshapen cartilage between the nostrils (see Nose). Less common is surgery to build up cheekbones or to alter a weak or oversize chin or jaw.

Rhytidectomy (a face-lift) will tighten the skin of the face when it starts to sag and wrinkle and will reduce a double chin if necessary. Puffy eyelids and bags under the eyes can be corrected by blepharoplasty (an eyelid-lift). Eyelid surgery is also done to lift drooping upper lids that may interfere with a person's eyesight. Ears that stick out, either because the middle part is too big or because the upper fold is badly formed, can be pinned back by otoplasty.

Skin scarred by acne, or disfigured by stretch marks or birthmarks, can be treated by dermabrasion, which rubs away the top layers of skin, or by chemosurgery (a chemical peel), which dissolves the surface layers with a form of acid (see Birthmarks). Thread veins or spider veins—harmless red marks caused by blocked capillaries near the surface of the skin—can be treated with laser therapy or sclerotherapy. Both treatments close off the veins, which then shrivel up (see Veins).

Cosmetic surgeons use synthetic implants to reconstruct breasts that are thought to be too small or are misshapen after injury or surgery. Breast reduction is sometimes done to relieve back and shoulder pain or breathing problems, as well as for cosmetic reasons. Mastoplexy (surgery that lifts drooping breasts) may be done at the same time as breast enlargement or reduction.

People with areas of fat that remain even after they have lost weight can have liposuction, a technique that removes fat by suction through a special tube. Fat concentrated in areas such as the stomach can be removed by lipectomy, a more serious procedure. This involves surgery to remove the fat and cut down and tighten any excess skin. A similar operation may be performed to reduce bags of skin left after rapid, extensive weight loss (see Surgery; Weight).

What is involved

Cosmetic operations may involve cutting and repairing flaps of skin and muscle; grafting an area of skin from another part of the body; removing or implanting cartilage, bone, or tissue; or implanting a synthetic substance. They range from simple treatments to major surgery requiring weeks of convalescence.

Because problems can arise with any kind of operation, a person should think carefully before deciding on cosmetic surgery. The surgeon should discuss exactly what the operation involves, including the hazards and recovery time, and should find out if the

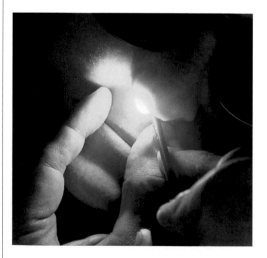

▲ *A surgeon uses a laser beam to remove superficial blood vessels around a patient's nose.*

Questions and Answers

I've been saving up to have the bags under my eyes removed by cosmetic surgery. Where should I look for a reliable surgeon?

The best way to find a surgeon is to get a recommendation from someone who has had successful surgery. Alternatively, your regular doctor may recommend one. Check with the American Board of Plastic Surgery to make sure that any specialist you go to is trained and accredited in this area.

I've tried dieting without much success, and I am tempted by the idea of liposuction. Is it the answer to my weight problem?

If you are overweight, liposuction will not solve your problem. This procedure works best on limited pockets of fat that do not respond to dieting. Lipectomy can yield better results, but it is not an alternative to eating less. Try to get down to your ideal weight first, because losing or gaining pounds afterward will distort the results of lipectomy. And surgery will not give you the health benefits of diet and exercise.

I'm planning to have my breasts enlarged, but a friend told me that silicon implants can cause breast cancer. Is this true?

The silicon gel filling of older breast implants sometimes leaks out. It was claimed that this could lead to autoimmune diseases (in which the body is attacked by its own defense system) but this is no longer believed to be true. This may be what your friend is thinking of. In any case, the Food and Drug Administration banned these implants for use in cosmetic surgery in the United States in 1992. Implants used now may be filled with harmless saline solution. Neither type of implant has been shown to increase the risk of breast cancer.

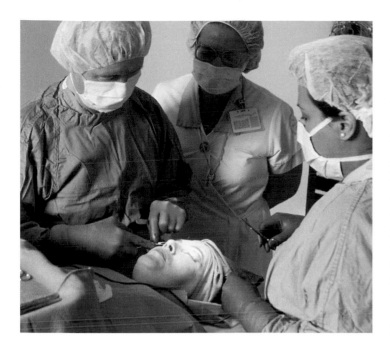

▲ A surgical team performs a cosmetic operation to reduce and tighten up the surplus skin on a patient's eyelids. Bags under the eyes can also be reduced.

prospective patient has any health problems that could increase the risks. It is important that the cosmetic surgeon does not encourage unrealistic expectations. Patients may be shown a computerized image that gives an impression of what they will look like after surgery, but this must not be taken as an exact guide.

Even simple surgical procedures can produce swelling and a bruised look for several days, and serious surgery requires weeks to recover from (see Bruises).

Rhinoplasty

Rhinoplasty may be done under a general or local anesthetic. The surgeon makes an incision, usually from inside the nostrils to avoid leaving obvious scars, separates the bone and cartilage that give the nose its shape from the tissue holding it together, and breaks the bone so that it can be set in a different shape. The cartilage may also be cut or shaved, or cartilage or bone from another part of the body may be implanted. Occasionally a synthetic implant is used. After the operation, the nose is stuffed with gauze, and it may also be held in shape with a splint for a week or two.

Breast enlargements and reductions

Breast enlargement may be done under a general anesthetic but often needs no overnight hospital stay. The surgeon makes a small incision, either under the breast or in the armpit. This enables him or her to insert an implant, or prosthesis, made of a synthetic pouch containing saline or silicon solution. This is tucked behind the breast tissue and muscles, pushing the tissue outward to make the breasts larger. The breasts may be sore and bruised-looking for a while after the operation, and there may be some loss of feeling for a time. The patient usually recovers normal feeling after healing. A woman's ability to breast-feed should not be affected (see Breasts).

Breast reduction is a more complicated and more drastic operation than enlargement. An incision like an upside-down "T" is made from the nipple downward and along the underside of the breast, and breast tissue is then cut away. In some cases the nipple and the areola, the dark ring around it, stay attached to the underlying tissue and are put back higher up on the breast; in other cases, a special skin graft is used in place of the nipple and areola. The patient will usually need to stay in the hospital overnight and will take several weeks to recover. She will not be able to breast-feed afterward if the nipple has been removed during the operation.

Removing fat and liposuction

Lipectomy to remove large areas of fat is another serious operation that usually needs at least an overnight stay in the hospital. The surgeon makes one or more incisions where the fat needs to be removed and loosens the skin and fat. Then he or she takes out the fat and cuts away any excess folds of skin. Sometimes, as with abdominal lipectomy (a stomach tuck), the surgeon will tighten the underlying muscle with stitches. He or she then sews the skin and tissues back together, leaving tighter skin and a slimmer shape.

A less severe technique that works on smaller areas of fat is liposuction, which is often done on an outpatient basis. The surgeon makes a small incision so that a cannula (a tube) can be inserted into the layer of fat and tissue between the skin and the muscle. Fat cells and liquefied fat are sucked out. The surgeon inserts the cannula through other incisions around the area, until the fat has been evenly reduced. He or she then sews up the incisions and covers the area with a tight dressing to reduce bruising. Liposuction may be performed with a lipectomy or may be done as part of a face-lift (see Liposuction).

Face-lifts

Face-lifts vary greatly, but in the basic technique the surgeon makes an incision at each side of the face, loosens the skin and fat from the muscles beneath, and trims away superfluous fat before pulling up and stitching the skin to leave a tauter surface. A face-lift may include a forehead, or coronal, lift, involving an incision under the hairline and an incision under the chin to reduce a double chin (see Plastic and Reconstructive Surgery).

Risks of cosmetic surgery

Some types of cosmetic surgery are more serious than others and so have more potential complications. However, all operations involve pain and the risk of bleeding, scarring, and nerve damage—causing short- or long-term damage to feeling and responses in the skin or muscles—as well as the dangers associated with anesthesia.

Infection is a risk when artificial implants are used, and antibiotics may be prescribed to counter this. Another problem with synthetic implants is that they do not wear as well as the human body and may need to be replaced after several years. Neither will operations to tighten skin and muscle last a lifetime; skin and breasts will eventually sag, thanks to a loss of elasticity and the action of gravity. The other risk is that of disappointment. While some people have their confidence boosted by cosmetic surgery, others may be disappointed if they find that reshaping their body has not solved their broader personal problems.

See also: Capillaries; Cartilage; Lasers; Muscles; Pain; Scars; Skin and skin diseases; Stomach; Stretch marks; Swellings; Wrinkles

Coughing

Coughing is not dangerous, or a disease, in itself. However, it may be an indication of something more serious. A respiratory infection will cause one type of cough, whereas smoking will cause another.

A cough is an explosive current of air driven forcibly from the chest. It forms part of a protective reflex to clear the air passages of any obstruction. Irritation of the upper airways by noxious gases and inflammation by infections cause coughing by a similar mechanism, but in this case the coughing is persistent.

Coughing is an essential protective mechanism designed to get rid of potentially harmful substances in the lungs and air passages. Using medicines to suppress a cough may do more harm than good (see Mucus; Phlegm).

Symptoms

The most important symptom is not the cough itself, but rather the material that is coughed up, the frequency of the coughing, and whether there is any pain. A persistent cough caused by smoking indicates low-grade chronic bronchitis (see Smoking). The person is in danger of developing COPD, lung cancer, and other disorders if he or she does not quit smoking (see Lung and Lung Diseases).

Coughs are not dangerous. However, exhausting coughs—accompanied by hoarseness, chest pains, breathlessness, fever, fatigue, and weight loss—should always be treated by a doctor.

In adults, a dry, persistent cough without any phlegm may be a symptom of pneumonia or heart disease, though an inflammation of the trachea (windpipe) or bronchi (the large air passages in the lungs) is more likely. If the cough is productive (produces phlegm) and the color of the phlegm changes from white to yellow or green, this is a sign of infection. In asthma without infection, the phlegm is white and frothy. Bloodstained phlegm may indicate lung cancer, pneumonia, or tuberculosis. Coughing that becomes painful can be a symptom of the development of pleurisy. In children, croup might be the cause of a cough with noisy, labored breathing that is dry and then produces mucus. Coughs that sound like crowing, with heavy phlegm, might be whooping cough.

Treatment and outlook

Diagnosis is based on phlegm color and the other symptoms. Antibiotic drugs may be given to treat certain infections (see Antibiotics). Bronchodilators are usually used to relieve asthma, and surgery may be necessary in cases of cancer (see Asthma). Stethoscope examination of the chest, possibly followed by an X ray, enables the doctor to determine the cause (see X Rays). Minor coughs will get better on their own.

See also: **Bronchitis; Chronic obstructive pulmonary disease; Hoarseness; Irritants; Pleurisy; Pneumonia; Pollution; Stethoscope; Tuberculosis; Whooping cough**

Questions and Answers

Do cough medicines really work?

Cough medicines do work in that they can suppress or stimulate a cough, but there is much debate about whether or not they are necessary. Cough syrups with codeine or dextromethorphan will suppress a cough. Specially formulated expectorants will help to dilute and loosen the mucus gathered in the mucous membranes of the respiratory system, making coughing easier. A hot drink with honey and lemon can be similarly soothing.

I coughed up yellow phlegm when I had a bad cold recently. Why?

Phlegm is normally clear mucus and indicates that the secretions of the mucous membrane are normal. If the color changes to either yellow or green, it implies that there is an infection present. Since this cleared up by itself in your case, it could not have been serious. For more serious infections, a visit to the doctor is necessary—he or she may prescribe a course of antibiotics.

Does coughing spread infection?

Yes. Although coughing and sneezing are reflex responses to outside stimuli, such as dust or gas, they can also transmit germs if a person has a respiratory infection. This is why it is so important to cover your nose or mouth and to avoid coughing or sneezing directly onto anyone.

Why is it that I sometimes can't control my coughing?

Coughing is the body's way of dealing with a foreign body in the upper airways or inflammation in the trachea. It is a reflex action—the messages to and from the brain are extremely rapid and not under voluntary control.

Simple cough remedies

SYMPTOMS	REMEDY
Postnasal drip (mucus dropping down from back of nose).	Ephedrine or similar drops, 3 or 4 times a day. See doctor after 5 days.
Inflammation of the back of the throat or larynx.	Inhalations of menthol or eucalyptus vapor, several times a day.
Irritating, throaty cough.	Cough lozenges.
Dry cough or cough interfering with sleep.	Cough syrup or suppressant. Take 2 teaspoonfuls, up to 3 times a day and at night.
Thick, sticky phlegm that will not come up easily.	Expectorant cough syrup, as directed on the bottle.

Cough syrup

Questions and Answers

I have some cough syrup left over from when I had a cough a few months ago. Is it still safe to use?

Although it is unlikely to do any harm, it is best to buy a new bottle, checking the expiration date. Generally, you should throw away medicines left over after an illness.

Is taking a honey and lemon mixture as good as taking a proprietary cough medicine?

Although a honey and lemon mixture is pleasant and soothing, it is doubtful whether this mixture can suppress the cough reflex, as cough syrups do. A medicine containing codeine or dextromethorphan would be much more effective, but only if taken on a doctor's advice.

Someone once told me that a cough syrup is a medicine that should be licked off a spoon. Is this the way it should be given?

In practice a cough syrup is often licked off the spoon because it may be too thick to run easily. Holding a cough syrup in the mouth for a few moments before swallowing is useful, to get the benefit of its soothing effect on the throat. Once it is swallowed, the active ingredients will be absorbed into the bloodstream.

Can I give my child cough syrup?

Yes, if you are sure that it is a cough which ought to be suppressed and that the constituents and dose of the cough syrup are safe in terms of the child's age and weight. There are many cough syrups that are made especially for children; these can be particularly helpful in dealing with a cough that is causing a child distress at night. Your doctor can advise you.

Many people incorrectly refer to any cough medicine as a cough syrup. In fact, a cough syrup is a particular type of medicine used to soothe and suppress coughs that are dry and irritable.

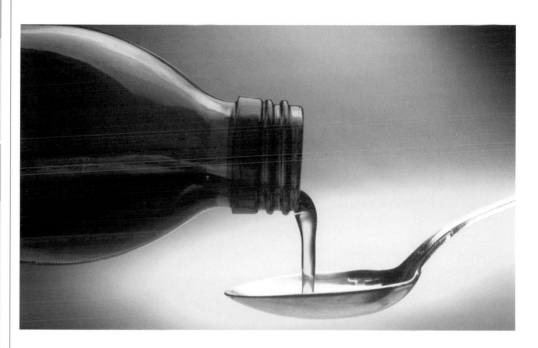

▲ *Suppressants such as cough syrups should be used only for nonproductive coughs.*

Cough syrups are sweet, sedative syrups, with a honey, molasses, or similar base, which suppress, or at least soothe, dry, irritable coughs. If a person has a cough, it is always wise for him or her to seek medical advice. The doctor can suggest the most suitable preparation to deal with that person's particular symptoms (see Breathing; Coughing).

Cough syrups come in varying strengths, depending on the active ingredients and the proportions in which they are made up. The most effective cough suppressants are morphine and methadone (physeptone), but these are used only for severe, unremitting coughs that occur in conditions such as advanced lung cancer. Less potent, but still effective, are cough syrups made from suppressants such as codeine or dextromethorphan.

Reasons for coughing

Coughing forces unwanted material, such as phlegm, out of the lungs and air passages so that it does not interfere with breathing or spread infection in the lungs. Therefore, when a cough is productive, it can be dangerous to use a suppressant because infected phlegm will stay in the lungs. Instead, an expectorant, which helps bring up phlegm, should be used (see Phlegm).

If the cough is dry and unproductive, causing pain and interfering with sleep, a cough syrup should be taken. However, if this dry cough arises from irritation at the back of the throat, as in pharyngitis (sore throat), then sucking a cough drop or lozenge may be more effective (see Pharynx; Sore Throat).

Cough syrup is usually taken in doses of two teaspoonfuls (0.34 fluid ounces, or 5 ml, each), up to three times a day and at night. Weaker preparations are suitable for children.

In some cases it is sensible to take an expectorant during the day and a cough syrup at night to quiet the cough and aid sleep.

See also: Emphysema; Expectorants; Infection and infectious diseases; Influenza; Lung and lung diseases; Medicines; Sedatives; Sleep and sleep problems; Symptoms; Throat

427

Counseling

Counseling is a way of helping people understand their problems and recognize and deal with their feelings. Through attentive listening and appropriate questioning, and sometimes by providing information, counselors enable people to find their own solutions to their problems.

Counseling is simply a formal way of having someone to talk to, but it is often more effective than just talking to a friend or relative. A trained counselor is able to listen in a more detached, unbiased, and honest way than someone who is involved in an individual's life, and the client has the reassurance that whatever is said is kept in complete confidence and will not be repeated.

Who it can help

An individual may feel that he or she would like to try counseling because of a specific problem in life, such as bullying, difficulties with other family members or the opposite sex, examination nerves, or just a general feeling of dissatisfaction or unhappiness. Counselors can also help at times of crisis: for example, the death of a loved one or rape.

Short-term counseling is sometimes provided when important decisions need to be made, such as whether to undergo a specific treatment at a hospital. In such cases the counselor will have specialized knowledge to help the person explore all the options. Counseling is also

Questions and Answers

What is the difference between counseling and psychotherapy?

Psychotherapists tend to treat deeper-seated problems than counselors, and they may delve into your distant past to find out about your childhood, or your internal world, and ask about your dreams and fantasies. In practice, however, there is considerable overlap between the two, and many counselors use psychotherapeutic techniques. Counseling can be short-term, and just one or two sessions can help you through a difficult time.

How can I be sure that nothing I say will be repeated elsewhere?

All counselors who belong to a professional body adhere to a strict code of ethics. This means that everything you say in a counseling session will be treated in confidence. However, if a counselor discovers that a murder or an act of terrorism has been committed, or is being planned, he or she must inform the police.

How do I find a good counselor?

Many schools, colleges, hospitals, and workplaces have counselors on the staff. Specialist bodies that deal with particular problems, such as drug and alcohol abuse, HIV/AIDS, interracial conflict, or family breakups usually have highly trained counselors. Private therapists can be found through your doctor, natural health centers, advertisements, or personal recommendations.

Is counseling expensive?

Counseling at school, college, or work may be free, but some organizations ask for voluntary contributions. Fees for private counseling vary; the most expensive is not always the best.

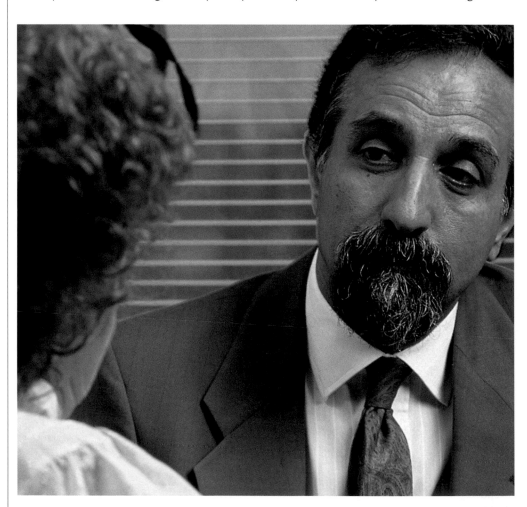

▲ *In a counseling session, client and counselor may sit quite close together. The counselor focuses his or her attention exclusively on the client and the client's problems.*

sometimes recommended for physical conditions that may have a psychological origin or be caused by stress, such as back pain or eating disorders. A person can be counseled alone, with a partner or other family members, or in a group.

Choosing a counselor

When counseling is provided as a service at a college, hospital, or workplace, it is not normally possible to choose a counselor. However, for long-term counseling it will usually be necessary to find a private therapist, and it is important to find the right person.

Counselors call the people that they see clients. Some counselors receive clients in their own homes; others have more formal premises elsewhere. Some will have a couch for the client to lie on; others, a comfortable chair to sit in. It is often up to the clients to decide what format suits them best and makes them feel relaxed. Some people prefer to keep a distance between themselves and their counselor; others prefer to be closer. The clients also need to decide what kind of counselor they will feel most comfortable with. Should he or she be the same sex—even the same race—a specialist, or someone used to dealing with more general problems?

Some counseling is done on the telephone. This is ideal for clients who want to preserve their anonymity, for people who are unable to travel, or when immediate support is vital—perhaps when someone is contemplating suicide.

Seeing a counselor

In long-term counseling, the first session is likely to be exploratory, with the client deciding whether this is someone he or she feels comfortable with, and the counselor assessing whether he or she can offer the kind of help the client needs. The client has nothing to lose at this stage by being honest and expressing any misgivings about the whole idea of counseling, about the counselor, or about anything else. The client may even find that this is the beginning of the unraveling process.

Counselors are trained to recognize serious mental problems, and if they think the client needs a different kind of therapy, they will say so immediately (see Psychology; Psychiatry). On the other hand, a counselor would never dismiss a client's problems or concerns as trivial. This would go against the whole ethos of counseling.

At the first session the counselor will also give the client an idea of how many sessions he or she thinks may be needed. Sessions are usually weekly, and counseling may extend over a few weeks or a year or more. The client need not decide at the outset how long the counseling will last, and sessions are usually paid for one at a time.

What counseling is like

A counselor gives the client his or her complete attention. This in itself is therapeutic—how many people have the luxury in daily life of being properly listened to? In addition, this attention is uncritical. A counselor is there not to judge clients but to help them understand themselves. When someone else really listens, the client starts listening to him- or herself.

The counselor may prompt the client with questions, if he or she feels that this is necessary. These are not the sort of questions that friends ask, which are usually motivated by curiosity, but questions designed to help the client see things more clearly. They may be questions no one has ever asked before or questions the client has never asked him- or herself. In family therapy the counselor's

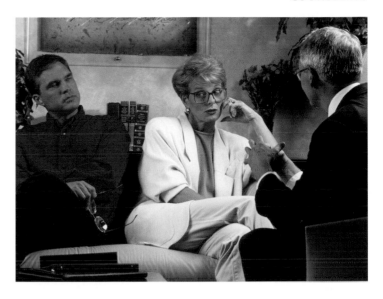

▲ *When partners are experiencing difficulties in their relationship, it can be helpful to discuss their differences with a third party who is a trained counselor.*

questions may induce family members to say things that other members of the family never knew they thought or felt. Another technique counselors use is "reflecting back" to clients the things the clients have said or feelings they have expressed or only hinted at. The counselor may say something like, "So, when this happens, you feel such and such, and this leads you to …." This not only shows that the counselor has heard and taken in what a client has said but makes the clients feel that they are being taken seriously and that their feelings have been given validity.

Release of emotion

In the course of counseling, the client may experience strong emotions—perhaps unexpected ones—and the counselor will encourage the client to explore and release these emotions. Because the counselor is not involved in the emotions, it is safe for the client to feel them without any risk of upsetting anyone or provoking anger in anyone. In partner and group sessions, a counselor can act as a sort of referee, turning emotional conflicts into constructive events that offer insights into the relationships. Some counselors offer physical contact at these times—holding hands or hugging, for example—but this is a matter of personal style.

The aim of counseling is to increase a client's confidence and make him or her more at ease with life in general, and to enable the client to be more in control of his or her own life.

What can go wrong?

There may be a few counselors who are not as professional as they should be. Some of the problems that might be encountered are:
● Physical contact that oversteps the bounds of what is acceptable.
● Breaches of confidentiality.
● A counselor who tries to dominate the client. If this is happening, the client will tend to feel worse after a session rather than better.
● A counselor who spends too much time talking about him- or herself. A certain amount of self-revelation is permissible in a counselor—it shows sympathy for what the client is saying—but this should be relevant and kept to a minimum.

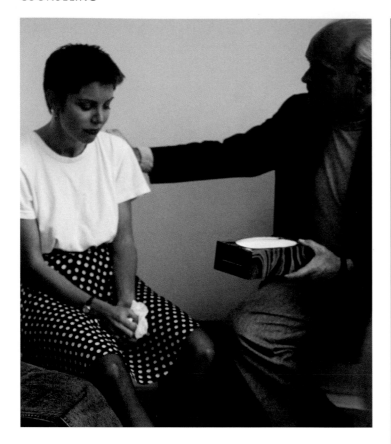

▲ *A client may find that strong and even surprising emotions emerge in him or her during a counseling session. However, counselors expect this to happen and are trained to sympathize with the client and to give him or her their support.*

• A counselor who wants too much social contact outside the sessions. Social contact changes the nature of the counseling relationship and is not usually a good idea.

When things go wrong

The first person a client should complain to is the counselor. Whether or not this is easy to do is in itself an indication of the health of the relationship between client and counselor. If the counselor works in an organization, such as a college, the client should discuss the problem with someone in authority. The professional organization the counselor belongs to can also be contacted. Serious offenses should be reported to the police, but it is wise in these circumstances to remember that it will be the client's word against the counselor's.

A bad experience should not be allowed to deter someone from finding another counselor. Most counselors are dedicated and skilled. However, dissatisfaction with the counselor may be a sign that the therapy is coming to an end.

Saying good-bye

The client is in charge of the course of the counseling and should always be the one to decide when to end it. Some people may need the support of a counselor all their lives, but this is highly unusual. The aim of counseling is to empower the client, not to make him or her dependent on another person, in this case the counselor. Some clinics allow only a limited number of sessions anyway. In short-term

Types of therapy

Cocounseling: In cocounseling, two people work together, taking turns as counselor and client. Both need to be trained to do this, but once trained, people can work in pairs to develop their own understanding of themselves, at the same time helping the other person.

Gestalt therapy: This is based on the belief that we all have an innate ability to function in a creative, positive, and healthy way but that social conditioning can impair this ability. The therapy uses techniques, such as reenacting arguments, to put you more in touch with your own emotions. It can be done either on your own or in a group.

Person (client)-centered therapy: This form of therapy aims to help people achieve their full potential. It is based on the belief that once people understand themselves better, they will be able to find their own way out of any difficulties they may have. The therapist relies less on theories and more on following what the client seems to want. The therapy was founded by U.S. psychologist Carl Rogers. Most counseling is based on person-centered therapy.

Psychiatry: The treatment of mental illness with drugs or surgery. Psychiatrists are medically trained.

Psychoanalysis: An intensive form of psychotherapy, often lasting several years, with several sessions a week.

Psychodynamic counseling: Counseling that uses psychotherapeutic techniques.

Psychology: The scientific study of the mind.

Transactional analysis: This was invented by Eric Berne, a Canadian doctor who believed that we have three ego states (ways of behaving): parent, adult, and child. Treatment aims to make people aware of which ego state they are in at any time and ultimately to express all three at once.

therapy the end will be in sight all through the counseling, and every counseling session will work toward this.

It is vital to finish counseling properly, so as not to undo what has been learned or devalue the whole process. There will be difficult emotions—anger that the counselor cannot help anymore, sorrow at the parting, fear that one cannot manage on one's own. All these emotions can be worked through in the final sessions.

Preparing to stop counseling can take several sessions. One way to prepare for an ending is to space counseling sessions more widely apart. The client can leave the door open at the final session: "I am leaving for now, but I can always come back if I need to." Some people return at times of stress throughout their lives.

See also: Abortion; AIDS; Alcoholism; Anorexia and bulimia; Child abuse; Drug abuse; Drug counseling; Family relationships; Grief; Stress management

INDEX

Index